HOW TO BE A PATIENT

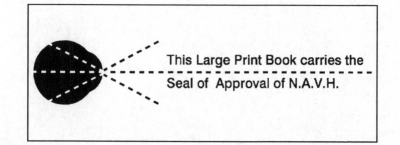

This Large Print Book carries the
Seal of Approval of N.A.V.H.

HOW TO BE A PATIENT

THE ESSENTIAL GUIDE TO NAVIGATING
THE WORLD OF MODERN MEDICINE

SANA GOLDBERG, RN

THORNDIKE PRESS

A part of Gale, a Cengage Company

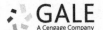

Farmington Hills, Mich • San Francisco • New York • Waterville, Maine
Meriden, Conn • Mason, Ohio • Chicago

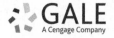

Thorndike Press® Large Print Lifestyles.
The text of this Large Print edition is unabridged.
Other aspects of the book may vary from the original edition.
Set in 16 pt. Plantin.

LIBRARY OF CONGRESS CIP DATA ON FILE.
CATALOGUING IN PUBLICATION FOR THIS BOOK
IS AVAILABLE FROM THE LIBRARY OF CONGRESS

ISBN-13: 978-1-4328-6380-7 (hardcover alk. paper)

Published in 2019 by arrangement with HarperWave, an imprint of HarperCollins Publishers

Printed in Mexico
1 2 3 4 5 6 7 23 22 21 20 19

For Tess, Mamie, and Gabe

CONTENTS

8

13

17

AUTHOR'S NOTE

For the purposes of this book, the terms "female" and male" generally relate to natal sex, or, the parts someone was born with. For reasons solely related to language clarity and anatomically relevant content, some verbiage is gender-specific. Content is written to be inclusive of individuals of all gender expressions and identities. This reflects a vacancy in adequate language and research in the medical field, but progress in the area is underway. See chapter 26 for specifics on transgender care.

Next, this table of contents is meant to serve as something of an index so that you can use this book as a field guide. It is both a tool and a story.

PREFACE

I was raised by an obstetrician who used to take me with her for weekend rounds. She was a single parent, and I was shy and bookish, never wanting to stray far from her orbit. It was a convenient arrangement.

She'd drop me at the nurses' station, where I'd help unload speculums from the sterilizer or write the names of new admits on the dry-erase board. I'd wander to the nutrition room, stocked with saltines and those little juice cups with foil lids. I'd stop by the nursery, and, transfixed, stand with new dads as we watched their plump newborns roll around in Lucite carts. Next to the nursery was a glorious standing linen warmer, where I'd take armfuls of blankets — which, if you've nuzzled into a pile of laundry straight from the dryer, you know the distinct pleasure of — and build forts or read *Little Women* in the call rooms.

I was fascinated by the swift order of

things, curious every time I saw someone whisked off to the OR . . . and plainly horrified to learn what a circumcision was! But I knew I liked this place, preferred it to home and certainly to school. The buzzing sense of purpose and the kindnesses exchanged planted memories that would yield a particular fondness for the world of medicine.

Because I'm still of an odd breed that feels at ease walking through badly lit, linoleum-floored hallways in scrubs and eating cafeteria food at insensible hours, here I am today. I've become a nurse. I've been a patient. I've watched both friends and strangers move in and out of the vast and complicated maze I used to play in. As children do, I perceived the world as uncharted territory and took joy in the process of understanding its convolutions. While the curiosity persists today, the romanticism has worn off, to say the least.

We speak often of the miracles of the world of modern medicine, and at its height it is miraculous indeed. But like all worlds, it has an underbelly, one you're likely familiar with if you picked up this book. The spaces we navigate in pursuit of our healthcare today can be confusing, chaotic, and defeating. A recent article stated, "In the 21st century, we still have to come to terms with the absurd reality that it is significantly safer to board a commercial airplane, a spacecraft, or a nuclear submarine, than to be admitted to a U.S. hospital."[1] An absurd reality that's difficult to reconcile, as most of us don't enter a hospital of our own accord. With alarming consistency, the purpose and order patients rely on when they enter the world of medicine is revealing itself to be uncomfortably tenuous.

It's interesting to come to love your profession while periodically losing faith in the way it functions. To be a nurse today is to tolerate the dissonance. It's to become acutely aware of the fractures in our medical infrastructure by witnessing things fall through them everywhere from community clinics to operating rooms.

Since becoming a healthcare professional, I've sat in on appointments where providers raced the clock and patients weren't able to say much of anything. I've listened to patients, in turn, tell me the intimate details of their concerns and expectations and then watched them fall silent and nod placidly when a team of white coats came into the room. I've seen medical error impact most people at some point, whether or not they knew it, and I've witnessed the insidious forms of racism and sexism that still affect how people receive care.

I faced these realities outside of my job as well. My grandfather died prematurely from misdiagnosis. My dad once sat in an ER with a pulmonary embolism and was told he was just tired and needed to go sleep it off! (In the chapter "When You're Having a Baby" we'll see how Serena Williams was ignored on this front, too.) My stepmom filed for bankruptcy because of ICU medical bills. My mother, the MD who used to tote me along to the hospital, underwent aggressive chemotherapy unnecessarily.

These challenges aren't limited to my family, of course. Since I've become a nurse, I've started to tune in when healthcare comes up in conversations out in the world. Whether it's with a Lyft driver, a friend, or a stranger — similar trends emerge. People are unsatisfied with their primary care provider. Often they don't have one. When they do show up for routine appointments, people say it's rare to feel listened to. Many instead tell of having their pain dismissed outright in a hospital (most patients facing this predicament are women, by the way, which we'll get to in "The Female Patient," page 469). These stories are typically accompanied by a collective air of disappointment and resignation.

The confusion, too, is universal. Whether recounting a series of appointments for a chronic illness, or a hospital stay, many struggle to reconstruct a narrative because the system struggles to explain things in a useful way. Other stories are more black and white, like a classic where the narrator goes to the ER for something minor (because it was a weekend and they didn't know where else to go) and leaves with a bill far exceeding their monthly income.

Some experience these adversities despite having access to care, and others because they can't access care to begin with due to the health inequities that pervade our society. We don't all enter the world of modern medicine from a level playing field, but the confusion doesn't discriminate. I've met college-educated adults who don't know which screenings are covered or when they're due. Highly organized and diligent individuals who are at a loss when it comes to navigating their aging parent's sudden hospitalization, especially dealing with a team of fifteen doctors at a teaching hospital.

So, no, these are not our glory days. The blame, then, flies off in multiple directions.

Some providers blame patients (burdening the system with unhealthy lifestyles). Patients certainly blame providers (too rushed, too greedy) or politicians (some want to give everyone healthcare, and others want to take it away). Everyone certainly blames the medical-industrial complex. These frustrations transcend our differences. We meet them with the same disappointment regardless of political affiliation or social standing or belief system. No matter who you are, when you're sick, you don't want to navigate a maze. What you want to do is nod to somebody and say take care of me and trust that they will.

To be sure, there are incredible individuals and organizations trying ardently to fix the broken aspects of the system and deliver better care, but the conversations are rarely public facing, or inclusive of patient input. They rarely address *how patients can advocate for themselves* in these highly challenging, precarious circumstances. In the moments I get a seat at the table, I ask why. *What can patients themselves do to counteract these forces?* The responses from practitioners, scholars, and administrators alike reveal a belief that the average patient can't understand or be expected to address these issues. It follows that despite our talk of patient-centered care and personalized medicine, we neither expect nor help patients to retain agency in action.

The most profit-driven institutions in the healthcare system, Big Pharma and the insurance industry, count on it remaining this way. Disempowered patients — whether incapacitated due to illness, or illiterate in matters of healthcare — enable them to make more money and reinforce the existing cycle. (This book isn't, however, strictly about the current state of the medical system and the myriad ways it's broken, and its purpose isn't to fearmonger. There are enough independent sources of that!)

On the other side, many of the protagonists of this story — those trying to change the medical system for the better — assume that those of us on the inside can fix it by ourselves. For patients, this means accepting moving at a snail's pace until the problems with the healthcare system sort themselves out.

In the meantime: How can patients advocate for better care on their own behalf? It's a working question I pose to the healthcare community at large, and one I attempt — with the thoughtful input of many patients and care providers — to answer in this book.

Ultimately, we will take a populist approach. If I am emphatic about one thing, it's that I believe in patient agency *more* than any other force in the healthcare system that stands to alter it. I believe in the notion that patients can take concrete steps to learn and act to change tired, ineffective dynamics and get better care — and they can do so more effectively and immediately than industry leaders can. Moreover, there are things patients, and *only patients,* can do for themselves to achieve better healthcare. For that reason this book is about, and for, *patients,* and by extension, you.

I'm a begrudging optimist, but I'm pragmatic, meaning that I fully accept that you and I might never see the world of medicine in the United States become whole and functional. At the same time, I'm certain each of us can take steps to better navigate a perilous terrain with our best interests in mind. We can find allies within it, take advantage of underutilized resources, seek out information that's not readily offered, and learn, in ways large and small, how to ensure that patient well-being is truly the core priority of each medical encounter.

The essential point about this guide is that it's different from others on the subject for the simple reason that I've been trained to think like a nurse, and nurses are the fulcrum of the healthcare industry.

In a TEDx talk in 2016, I told Harvard undergraduate students that they should consider becoming nurses, taking their freshly signed diplomas and rigorous training in the sciences and humanities to a field commonly thought of as vocational. This is because, after patients, I believe nurses are best poised to change the future of healthcare.

Today, registered nurses spend more time physically present with patients than any other healthcare professional, and as a consequence we see and hear a lot. We maintain a vantage point markedly different from that of the MD, the scholar, the journalist, and the policy maker. We are intimately familiar with the complexity and multiplicity of the patient experience, as well as the systems in healthcare that fail to acknowledge it. We witness the system's barriers regularly, and in turn we come up with creative solutions to sidestep its most vexing realities.

Donna Diers, former dean of the Yale University School of Nursing, and Claire Fagin, former dean of the University of Pennsylvania School of Nursing, describe the profession as one born of the "indifference to power for its own sake . . . the pleasure associated with helping others from the position of a peer rather than from the assumed superordinate." They said it well. Nurses prefer to be shoulder to shoulder with our patients, looking at the problems laid out before us, creating a plan together.

Voted the most honest and ethical professionals in public Gallup polls every year (except in 2001, when they lost to firefighters), nurses are a bastion of trust in a system that invites a lot of mistrust. It follows that when you're a nurse, people like to tell you things. You become a vessel for stories, and you learn how to listen. Whether someone I meet at a party launches into telling me about their yeast infection, or their pursuit of a diagnosis, or the injustices of their recent hospital stay, the walls between public and personal, professional and civilian, readily subside. This trust and connection is a privilege, and it is not lost on me that it's what allowed this book to come to fruition.

I don't talk much about the work of nursing directly in this book, something that became evidently clear to me upon finishing it. But I privilege nursing as an organic consequence of my own experiences in healthcare. Every aspect of this book was shaped by the work and theory of nursing, in which patient advocacy and empowerment is a foundational principle. I hope this book is a testament to that way of thinking, and to the work of my colleagues, who are out in the field this very moment as I sit at a library carrel. I hope that reading this book prompts you to turn to the nurses around you with a new spirit of collaboration and understanding.

Last, and most important, this book is a field guide. It's not diagnostic, or prescriptive, or absolute. It doesn't go in depth into any one disease but lays out general truths and tools one can use when seeking care, young or old, sick or well. It's called an essential guide, but in truth you are the guide.

Self-help and how-to books make me a bit nervous when they say outright that if you follow steps A, B, and C, things will work out swimmingly. I'm wary of anything giving the impression that its solutions to complex issues are simple and instant, so long as you retain all the information and act on it as directed. This book doesn't work like that — not because changes won't result; they will — because the content of this book doesn't have to be retained in one fell swoop. Perhaps the most pernicious aspect of the modern healthcare system is that patients often resort to dealing with it when their defenses are at their lowest. Traversing the healthcare sector is daunting for anyone, but especially for someone whose emotional, physical, or financial reserves are depleted. This book attempts to initiate one major paradigm shift in the existing healthcare industry — that patient agency is integral to better healthcare — but beyond that, it can be read in pieces and returned to at various points along the care continuum, throughout life. Read it at your own pace, and implement these suggestions as you see fit. I hope it serves you as a lifelong companion.

■ ■ ■ ■

PART I
WHEN ALL IS WELL

■ ■ ■ ■

These opening chapters will discuss the golden rule on which this book is founded: Patient agency in the world of modern medicine is of paramount importance. But before we delve into navigating that world, I'll start with how most of us learned how to be a patient. And then promptly ask you to unlearn all of it.

ONE:
WHERE TO START

If you ever saw the film adaptation of Roald Dahl's *Matilda* as a kid, you probably haven't forgotten the scene where Matilda — and all of us desperately rooting for her — are hit with some cold, hard truths about being at a power disadvantage:

"I'm big and you're small, I'm right and you're wrong. There's nothing you can do about it."

Has being a patient ever made you feel, like Matilda, on the wrong end of this equation?

A power dynamic is consistently at play when healthcare encounters go south. It's often the culprit behind misdiagnosis, patient dissatisfaction with medical professionals, and disjointed, minimally helpful care to patients in emergencies or struggling with chronic illness. It's a reason some people avoid the healthcare system at all costs, and, on the extreme end of the spectrum, it contributes to medical error and death from preventable illness.

It boils down to this: *You tell me what's wrong, I tell you what to do.* It's an exchange that implies hierarchy and a one-way street. *I have, you need. I know, you don't.*

This is the model we've been given: that patients are passive recipients of care. It's a model that's been reinforced by messages we've internalized since we were kids.

From a young age, we learn that there's an agreed-upon role we play as patients. Simultaneously, we learn about social codes, and that there are some people in society we don't question. Most of them have uniforms so we can identify them more easily — police officers, doctors, priests — and basic ground rules apply to their station: You don't run from a cop, you don't curse at a priest, and you don't question a doctor. This white-coat syndrome, which we'll get to in the next section, affects us well into adulthood. Research has shown that most of us aren't even aware of its impact. Outside of this, we aren't taught how to be a patient. We don't learn in school, and it's not a practice we're set up to integrate into our lives like we might with yoga or healthy eating. We lack a model to becoming literate in matters of healthcare, or adept at navigating them. All of it adds up to a misguided message: that a patient's role begins and ends with being compliant.

Our expectation for providers, in turn, is that they are to be infallible. We expect them to produce the right solution, at the right time, every time, for what ails us. Our opinion of them is primed to be so high that at times we not only relinquish power but even exclude from the realm of possibility that they could make mistakes.

With simple things like stitches and yeast infections, this model works. It's fine! We can walk in with a standard problem, get assessed, receive a diagnosis, and walk out cured or headed to Walgreens. But many medical encounters are more nuanced. The source of symptoms is rarely obvious, their solutions could come from multiple directions, and whether the course of action is right largely depends on communication, shared agency and shared decision-making.

Compounding all of this is today's badly behaving, dysfunctional medical-industrial complex, in which the passive patient model increasingly leads to trouble — even when the problems are simple. Like all systems that ride on capitalism, its power is primed to be extreme and unrelenting, and its endgame is never your well-being.

At some point or another, each of us butts up against this model when we are subject to its flaws. For some, it happens when something more complicated than a cold arrives at their doorstep. For others it's a reality well before that, due to barriers that make quality care out of reach for many people in our society. This reckoning might come after an appointment, when you realize you have no idea as to the plan moving forward. Or when you're suddenly not sure if that appointment solved a problem or created new ones. For some, it comes with acquiring debt, or with realizing they were never fully informed about the risks of a procedure. The moment doesn't discriminate based on income, culture, or state of health. It comes for all of us, and it's universally defeating.

Instead of putting a fire under patients to tip the scales, assert agency, and partner with their providers, this reckoning usually — and understandably — leads to surrender. Have you felt disappointed when you couldn't get a diagnosis, or sheer fury when screwed by an insurance carrier? Have you thought: *I'm powerless and at a disadvantage, and it's clear to everyone and completely unfair?* And then later, when you're really tired or really sick, thought, *Well, this is how it is. What am I going to do? Not try to get better? Give up?* And so you keep enduring the same injustices, because you need healthcare. This is rational, and you're not alone.

Robb Willer, Stanford professor of sociology, calls this phenomenon the powerlessness paradox. In a social system like medicine, feelings of power determine whether people take on systemic oppression. When we feel powerful, we are more likely to oppose and act out against systems that oppress us, but, paradoxically, feelings of powerlessness cause us to support the existing order. Even when it's putting us at a disadvantage, and even as we're keenly aware of medicine's limitations — as we see disease win out, or learn men receive superior care to women.

Siddhartha Mukherjee frames the problem as a "queasy pivoting between defeatism and hope." The phrase, in its original context, is used to describe our fragile, tenuous relationship with a cure for cancer, but it lends itself to describing the balancing act required of all patients. It's the unrest that comes from depending on an imperfect process or system.

To be sure, this queasy pivoting, and the surrendering, is not reserved for patients.

Your providers know it intimately. Some might be just as scarred by the system as you are, while others find ways to provide excellent care despite it. It's my belief that the qualities that lead people to the healthcare profession — compassion, curiosity, empathy, a genuine desire to help others — still burn intensely in the people across from you at appointments, but for many they become casualties of the system. The powerlessness paradox is at play here too.

Medical providers do, of course, hold lots of power as well. And for good reason! They spent their golden years in the library, hospitals, and clinics learning how to heal us. It takes highly specialized training and a devotion to medicine to learn how to deliver a breach baby, excise a brain tumor, or reset a bone. That said, you'll have to step up to help them best wield it. A provider's license to practice medicine does not mean that they know you or your body best. They will come to better decisions about how to use their expertise if you meet them in making decisions about your health.

A sage doctor once told me there's no worse transgression in medicine than doing something for a patient *you* decide is helpful, while not taking into consideration whether or not *they* find it helpful, only to learn it's not, in fact, helpful. There's a word for this in German, *Verschlimmbessern,* which literally means "to improve for the worse" or, as my friend in Berlin translated for me, *"worse-better."* In a system where one in four people receives excessive or unwanted medical treatment, it's a term that's alive and well.

You cannot graduate from nursing school without hearing over and over again that your job is to meet people *where they are: that you treat a patient, with a disease, in the context of a lived life.*

We can't be diagnosed and treated in a Petri dish. Disease is never just its symptoms. It manifests in context, which is made up of lots of factors — our mental health, our environment, our socioeconomic status, our race, our gender, our temperament, our educational level, our age, our family history, our mood when we walk into a clinic. What our world looks like the 99.9 percent of time that we aren't in an exam room. All these things make up a patient. It means an identical disease, risk factor, or symptom could look different in each person, and the best course of action to address it should be personalized.

Medical encounters, when they're rushed,

tend to gloss over details about family history and mental health. They run the risk of omitting important questions, such as how much pain a patient feels they can live with, how they define quality of life, or how well they understand their disease. These are relevant, as later chapters will point out, in making decisions that are not black-and-white — for instance, whether quality or quantity of time is more important to you. To have another round of chemotherapy or not. To proceed with a risky operation or wait and see. These all rest on context. In the first and most important act of agency, patients have to assume responsibility for conveying this context. Otherwise, providers will infer, assume, or base decisions on Jane, the simulated robot patient they worked with in school.

PATIENT POWER IS ULTIMATE

In a study where patients were asked about their healthcare preferences . . . a lot of people started their answers with the words "Well, if I had a choice . . ."

And when I read that "if," I understood better why one in four people receives excessive or unwanted medical treatment, or watches a family member receive excessive or unwanted medical treatment.

It's not because doctors don't get it. We do. We understand the real psychological consequences on patients and their families. Half of critical care nurses and a quarter of ICU doctors have considered quitting their jobs because of distress over feeling that they've provided care that didn't fit with a person's values. But doctors can't make sure your wishes are respected until they know what they are.

— DR. LUCY KALANITHI

You have a choice at every turn. This is the next thing to take to heart.

Like Kalanithi, I often hear friends and family, exasperated by their healthcare experiences or struggling with unresolved illness, say:

If I could have known that beforehand
If I could have made this decision earlier
If I could have told my doctor "no"
If I could have pressed the issue further

You can. To break down the power dynamic, it's essential to realize this. Patients don't hear it enough for it to hit home, and even when they do hear it, they have trouble believing it.

One of the greatest mental shifts required is to realize that providers are there to counsel you through decisions — *not* make

43

them on your behalf or, worse, act with such authority as to imply there are no decisions to be made.

The goal of a medical encounter is to navigate health choices with your provider, who should inform and guide you through various options but should never dictate. The goal is to exchange what you both know and come to a decision together.

The final piece of the groundwork is realizing that as a patient, your power is ultimate.

When I was working in an acute mental healthcare setting, a patient case once caused a big stir around the nurses' station. The patient himself wasn't the problem — it was the logistics of his discharge. In the hospital, a lot of folks (providers, social workers, pharmacists) have to check their piece off in order to clear a patient to go. Sometimes this takes a wildly long time, with lots of opportunities for derailment.

That morning, the issue was a prescription. The patient had to have it before he got on the bus, but the on-call physician hadn't signed off on it, so the pharmacy was late getting it and the patient was going to miss his ride. The nurse and social worker were aggravated, but finally, much later and after the plan was altered significantly, the med came through.

I happened to be on break, eating my lunch outside across from the bus stop, when the patient walked out. He tossed the bottle of pills in the garbage bin, along with the paperwork on the follow-up appointments they'd scheduled for him, and hopped on the bus.

I'm a nurse, so of course I don't advocate tearing up your discharge paperwork or tossing your pills, but let this bold guy be a reminder that you never have to do anything. You can walk out, say no, wait and see, or find someone else and start over. It's not always this simple, because sometimes when you're sick, exhausted, or dependent on immediate care you don't have the option of starting over without making things worse. But your mentality can affect how small things within your treatment play out. Remind yourself, often, that as a patient your only obligation is to yourself.

One last bit to empower you: In research that explores how people use the medical system, patients are referred to as "consumers." Remember this! Remind yourself of it all the time. Patients are paying customers. *You* are a paying customer. Before you splurge on something on Amazon, you probably read the reviews. If a dress you ordered doesn't fit or the dish brought to your table is not what you ordered, you send it back! You don't permit stores to sell you things you don't need or didn't bring to the register. (We'll discuss how this happens in the medical world, and how to fend it off, in the section "Healthcare Bluebook.") For now, keep in mind that the rules on consumerism apply to medicine too.

Two:
Unlearn What You Know About Being a Patient

Before we delve in, a few subconscious obstacles to asserting agency during a medical encounter — and how to shed them.

Why I Use the Term "Provider"

I see red when I hear someone default to "he" and "doctor" as the universal nouns for people who practice medicine. It is antiquated and unhelpful to modern patients.

My insistence on using the term "provider" in this book isn't just to avoid cluttered sentences, but also to try to resolve a larger issue with the way words and titles impact and reinforce social constructs. In today's medical system, these constructs reproduce inequality and get in the way of care.

Let me explain how: A quick Google image search of the term "doctor" will yield predominantly men. There aren't many women to be found. But type in "nurse," and there are plenty. You don't have to scroll far before the stuff of sexy Halloween costumes pops up. Our perceptions of medicine are deeply gendered, based on an underlying attitude toward nurses and doctors that is at its core a stereotype.

So it's not hard to see why we default to "he" and "doctor" when referring to a hypothetical provider. It seems benign enough, but the language fails to challenge a deeply ingrained belief that when we are sick, we seek help from men in white coats. Our linguistic defaults devalue 34 percent of the physicians in our country (the female ones). And when we use the term "doctor" for anyone who oversees our healthcare, we erase fields of professionals who today serve care roles interchangeable with those of physicians.

A variety of types of medical professionals are providers, because they diagnose, prescribe, and direct a course of care with their patients. Some common providers include:

Physician, doctor: MD (doctor of medicine) or DO (doctor of osteopathic medicine)
Nurse practitioner: NP (nurse practitioner) or APRN (advanced practice

registered nurse)
Physician assistant: PA

"Provider" can function as a catchall label for these different roles.

Medicine can be seen as an interprofessional sport, in which nurses, pharmacists, therapists, and social workers among others are positioned to offer solutions and allay frustrations just as physicians are. Retraining yourself to see healthcare this way is critical to getting better care. There are always sources of support in our peripheral vision, people who can rise to the challenge and help, regardless of the letters after their name.

WHITE-COAT SYNDROME

The white coat, imbued with authority and prestige, is a powerful article of clothing. Civilians feel more intelligent and capable when they slip into one, and several studies show many of us prefer that our providers wear one. When someone dons a white coat we take them more seriously, feel we are in more knowledgeable hands, and unconsciously slip into a role of obedience.

If you ever took an intro to psychology course, it's likely you heard tales of the Milgram experiment. In 1961, shortly after the trial of Nazi war criminal Adolf Eichmann began in Jerusalem, Yale professor Stanley Milgram began what would become a seminal psychological study that attempted to quantify authority. His experiments involved a "teacher," a "student" in an electric chair, and an experimenter in a lab coat. The participant, always given the role of the "teacher," was told to shock the student if they answered questions incorrectly. With each incorrect answer, the participant was told to increase the voltage, assured by the experimenter in the lab coat that it didn't hurt the student.

This was all staged — no one was actually being harmed — but the participant didn't know this. The study found that the participant would continue to administer shocks despite staged cries and pleas from the recipient — even despite being informed that the recipient had a heart condition. The figure in the lab coat would say, "Keep going, you must continue" — and they did. (Milgram tapped into the power we assign to a lab coat, and consequently into our innate response to authority — showing that it's a universal tendency.)

Infer what you will about our moral character, but something happens when we register a white coat, and the effect dates back centuries. Into the late 1800s, doctors wore black. They were considered charlatans, thought to prattle and quack about town. In an effort to rebrand, they donned the white coats worn by scientists, whose reputation was on the ascent during the Industrial Revolution. Doctors went on to perform lobotomies, decide vibrators cured hysteria, perform cigar-smoke enemas, dole out cocaine drops for children's toothaches, and use mercury to clean wounds — all in white coats. Christiaan Barnard, the heart surgeon we'll discuss in chapter 7, struck up a side business with Clinique La Prairie in Switzerland, where he developed "rejuvenation" therapy using injections of extracts from sheep fetuses.[1] All the while, like others of his ilk, in a lab coat.

These micro-lessons in history teach us that we can't discount the powerful and unconscious influence of the white coat. We see it, and we take a back seat. We trust, we nod, we feel honored and privileged to be in its presence.

This influence can quell our instinct to question, speak up, or challenge a plan that was set in motion without our full understanding. It's the reason one in four people receives unwanted medical treatment, and the reason we're inclined to please providers and averse to disappointing them.

As they say in French, *"L'habit ne fait pas le moine"* — the robe does not make the monk — and *"la barbe ne fait pas le philosophe"* — the beard does not make the philosopher. The white coat is simply that — an article of clothing. (By the way, these coats harbor disease! Studies have found that their sleeves are prone to carrying MRSA and other microbes, scattering them around rooms and between patients.)

The boy who picked his nose in your third-grade class? He's probably off somewhere wearing one, a patient listening to his advice with bated breath.

PARADIGM SHIFT: FROM REACTION TO PREVENTION

The next important mental shift: Start thinking of healthcare as *preventive* rather than *reactive.*

Many illnesses and health emergencies are unavoidable, and no amount of planning or preparing will stave them off. However, those aren't the majority of what sends us to the health system. Studies have confirmed that of the five leading causes of premature death in the United States — cancer, heart disease, stroke, respiratory disease, and unintentional injury — 20 to 40 percent in each category are preventable.

It's completely understandable if you avoid seeking medical attention out of frustration or fear. But routine medical care is essential for preventing disease across life, and receiving the best routine care takes facing the music. It takes interfacing with the world of medicine, and it takes a little investment. To go without established care can catch up with you and make life harder. It will make dealing with certain medical problems more time-consuming and expensive than it has to be. If you've ever sat in an ER waiting room with a non–life threatening (but really uncomfortable) medical problem because you didn't know where else to get help, you know what I mean.

Avoiding preventive care can also cause economic burden. While routine appointments might seem financially inaccessible, going without that care can lead to even more expensive medical problems down the road as you age. (In the section "Getting Care When You're Uninsured," you'll find ways to obtain many preventive services for free without insurance.) Part of establishing routine care is planning for and preventing these burdens.

It takes time to build relationships, familiarize yourself with resources, and understand medical culture. But when you miss out on these steps, dealing with problems only as they arise, you constrict the planning and art of being a patient. Coming chapters will provide tools for taking advantage of screenings, tests, checkups, and relationships to get the most out of routine care, but simply this mental shift from reaction to prevention will take you a long way to better health throughout your life.

ADOPT RITUALS: THE ART OF BEING A PATIENT

My stepmother is the type of person who moves through the world with such ease and capability that it's impossible not to try, or at least wish, to emulate her. If there's a secret to living well, she's figured it out.

To describe her as merely "capable" doesn't quite do her justice, but it's fitting. She lives on black coffee, fruit, and champagne; speaks multiple languages; builds houses from the ground up; tells men what to do before they open their mouth to tell her; and cooks meals for herself with a thoughtfulness typically reserved for hosting dinner parties.

She's staunchly capable of doing anything she sets her mind to, on the condition that she enjoys it. And I don't mean she only

54

does things she wants to do, when she wants to do them. It's quite the opposite: She sees each challenge as something that will accommodate her joy in return for her efforts, if she gives herself to it and sees it to completion. Her experiences give her what she asks of them.

My boot-camp-style immersion in her ways came one summer when I had less than a month to sell my house, pack my things, and move across the country to start graduate school. She arrived at my doorstep and within two weeks packed all my belongings (save the dog and his food) into a portable storage unit and mapped out a road trip. We sold the house with the help of her baking, which sent tantalizing clouds of the scent of fresh-baked cookies past the open-house sign and into the streets to lure potential buyers in.

It's said that an epic move takes a toll that's comparable to a death in the family — packing, organizing, parting with things and people. I dreaded these tasks to my core, approaching the whole affair with aversion. But with my stepmother, the experience felt more like a party. She insisted there was enough time to accomplish our tasks efficiently, and there always was. We made a surplus of good memories

— ones I've bottled up and stored away for inspiration when a task feels insurmountable. We found a stride and celebrated achieving little goals. Somehow, we always found time to cook on each one of those summer nights, finish our books, and go for walks.

My stepmother does not lecture or teach (except on pragmatic subjects, like why to invest in a pressure washer). When it comes to the enlightened way she moves through the world, you just have to absorb it through osmosis.

One thing I've picked up on over the years is that she is a woman of rituals. The most contagious one, which I've adopted and passed on to friends, is the tradition of Champagne Sundays. A Champagne Sunday is just housekeeping — elevated. It's a half day or so dedicated to dusting, Swiffering, and taking care of the week's put-off chores, but with a spin involving champagne and speakers up to the challenge of blasting Fleetwood Mac. Of course, the bubbles and the music make the tiresome affair a bit rosier, but it's more the intentional framing that makes it work.

These days I never think, *Damn, I really need to spend time getting on top of this house.* Instead I think, *A Champagne Sun-*

day is in order.

This can also apply to taxes. I know a woman who, each year, cozies up on the couch and commences doing her taxes while she watches the Academy Awards. She's never bored during commercial breaks, she gets it out of the way early, and she's started actually looking forward to the whole ordeal.

Another friend's father taught her when she was little that washing dishes by hand was a privileged opportunity to practice zen. To this day, she insists on doing the dishes at my house every time she comes over.

Renowned Harvard psychology professor Ellen Langer showed the impact of mind-set through a study of hotel maids. She divided eighty-four maids into two groups: In the first cohort, researchers carefully went through the tasks the maids did each day and explained how many calories they burned, pointing out the myriad ways the maids' work was a form of exercise that met the surgeon general's recommendations for daily activity. The other group went about their tasks without the commentary from the researchers. Astonishingly, the study found that after several months, the maids in the first group experienced weight loss, decreased waist-to-hip ratio, and a 10 percent drop in blood pressure — just through the new mind-set that their jobs were physically good for them.

No one particularly loves or is enthusiastic about dealing with their healthcare. But if mind-set can literally change your metabolism and alter the way your body lays down fat cells, it can certainly make something unpleasant feel solidly good. It's the Champagne Sunday idea at work.

We can use the idea of mind-set to dramatically reframe the way we approach being a patient, from the way we greet the tasks of scheduling appointments and getting flu shots, to dealing with insurance companies.

Couch healthcare tasks with personal indulgences. Add a sparkling incentive to achieving goals. Approach the job with friends and partners. Like the work of gardening, or making the bed, or setting up the coffee pot the night before — ritual feels good. It is a task up front, and a gift later.

Nuisance to Ritual

You can look away when a medical bill arrives or work yourself into a conniption fit as you navigate the financial portion of your care — or you can use the experience to squeeze a little more delight into your month while checking things off your list.

Set aside one evening a month to review your insurance claims and status. Collect any Explanation of Benefits (EOB) forms, bills from therapists' offices or hospitals, and statements about eligibility and open enrollment. Put them in a pile on the table in front of you, or collect them digitally on your screen. Highlight and note things that are unclear, or items for which you need to gather more information from your insurance company. It's a chance to review everything in a low-stress setting, rather than randomly opening a claim after a long day of work and trying to ensure that there aren't any glaring issues. If your bill of health has been complicated as of late, set aside additional time to review upcoming appointments, tests, and procedures for which you'll eventually be charged. Most months this will be a pretty low-key task, one you can do while having a cold beer or watching a favorite show in the background. You can also make an outing and do it at a coffee shop.

Carve out time to call your insurance company. If you feel like overachieving, you can call them the same evening you do your review, or give them a call the following day. Many companies have limited hours, so you may need to call during work or other scheduled activities, but many do take calls outside the hours of nine to five.

Find friends or neighbors in the same boat (this may be easier than you think). If you or someone you provide care for has frequent encounters with the medical system, have a potluck or dessert hour. Brew a pot of coffee and dedicate an hour where everyone can work through their insurance papers. It's nice to be at a table together, with support for a task that can be depleting when faced alone. Tips and tricks of the trade will inevitably surface around the table.

Dangle a carrot for yourself. When something must be dealt with right away, like determining coverage for a procedure (see "Healthcare Bluebook," page 526), pick a reward, like going to a movie alone, taking a bath with fancy salts and oils, or opening the good wine.

INCREASE YOUR HEALTH LITERACY

Me: Dad, how's your health?
Dad: It's great. Tomorrow I'm going to see
my gynecologist.

— LISA FITZPATRICK MD

Have you ever glazed over as a provider started speaking Medical Encyclopedia, snapping back to attention at: *Any questions?* Pretended to understand something because you felt too intimidated to ask a question, or agreed to take a medication or follow a protocol, but not really understood why you're supposed to? If so, you're not alone. Something about the medical encounter makes us want to appear competent, and there's a commonly held belief that medical knowledge is (or should be) common knowledge. That everyone else besides you knows where the pancreas is, or what diuretics do, or what hypertensive means.

One of my own patients recently described being in a hospital as akin to being in another country. Studies indicate that 88 percent of the US population lacks sufficient health literacy, and the deficit is not only linked to confusion but to poorer health outcomes.[2] Health literacy has to do with how you read a pill bottle and decide on a dose, how well you understand a normal blood pressure range, how you respond when you run out of a medication. When individuals don't have access to health information in a form they can understand, it impacts all of these things, including how they navigate insurance, fill out complex forms, and assess risks and benefits of treatments. For the majority, navigating healthcare is not entirely different from trying to follow a recipe written in another language.

When patients walk out the door of their provider's office without a solid understanding of the exchange or the plan, they do not get a full opportunity to understand the intricacies of their disease and how to manage it out in the real world. Some avoid seeking medical care in the first place because it's demoralizing. I've had patients tell me outright they skip appointments because they know they'll be handed a clipboard of paperwork and they don't read well. Social determinants such as race, age, education level, and income bracket are correlated with health literacy, however, it's a barrier to care for people of all walks of life and educational backgrounds.

Ultimately, it's a matter of patient empowerment. There is a chasm between what providers know, and what patients can and need to understand. Some providers traverse it more elegantly than others. There are national efforts to improve the way clinicians attend to matters of health literacy, but in the meantime there are two aspects to achieving better health literacy that you can address yourself.

Improving Your Health Literacy Before You Have a Specific Health Situation on Your Hands

This section exists within "When All Is Well," because there are specific ways to give yourself a boost in the health literacy department before you need it. The first step involves dictionaries.

When it occurred to me that you don't have to be a nurse to use a nursing reference, I started telling friends and family to download the two apps I used most frequently in nursing school: the Farlex Nursing Dictionary and Epocrates.

The Farlex Dictionary allows you to quickly find the definition of any medical term that could possibly be tossed around. As it's meant to be something nurses can use on-the-go at the hospital or clinic, the interface is exceptionally simple. You just enter a word and it populates a short definition followed by additional information if you choose to keep scrolling.

I use the Epocrates app for medications. Accurate and comprehensive, it allows you to look up all drugs, including over-the-counter medications like Zyrtec and Advil, and easily find what they're taken for, what they do in the body, their different names, and their interactions with other drugs. The app will also tell you what type of patient isn't a good candidate for taking the drug (for instance, someone over sixty-five), and the most magical feature: it allows you to enter in the shape, color, scoring, and imprint of any pill and it will identify the drug for you.

If you prefer not to use your smartphone for yet another thing, or if, like me, you have an affinity for paper dictionaries, there are great equivalents! *Taber's Medical Dictionary* is a classic and one of my favorites, and the *Davis Drug Guide,* another nursing go-to, comes in a pocket-sized version that's easy to tote around.

Next, because health literacy is about competency and not just language, prepare yourself in basic first aid. Created by the American Red Cross, the First Aid App puts information about what to do in medical emergencies at your fingertips. Everyone should have it and peruse it now and then for muscle memory.

In addition to the resources outlined above, including information on what to do in emergency health situations and how to relay questions to providers which will come below, know that virtually every aspect of this book was designed with health literacy in mind. *The Patient's Guide to Health Literacy* didn't sound quite as fun as *How to Be a Patient,* but you get the gist. Consider this book a graduate level course on the subject!

Advocate for Yourself During Appointments to Ensure You're Getting Useful Information

The pearl here is to ask questions. And plow through any of the barriers (both those you impose on yourself and those imposed by the system) that prevent you from doing so. This topic is of such importance there's an entire chapter dedicated to it to come, but for now just remember to ask boldly and frequently, knowing you're in the company of most adults everywhere when you don't understand something.

Be an Upstreamist

The 1983 biographical film *Silkwood* tells the story of workers in a plutonium factory in the American South who start to develop various cancers and other health problems. One by one they drop like flies, as the plant owners hide any trace of the diseases' connection to the work environment. Meryl Streep plays Karen Silkwood, the film's heroine, who becomes a nuclear whistle-blower after realizing she and her colleagues are being exposed to copious amounts of radiation.

Work hazards, living conditions, geographic exposures, and life stressors are real determinants of health. There's an old tale that if you're a provider and hundreds of people from your town start coming in with diarrhea, you can give out prescription after prescription for antibiotics, or you can ask what the hell's in the water.

Rezoning laws and rent increases can cause chronic inflammation. Institutional racism and toxic stress can cause low birth weight. Exposure to air pollution can affect inflammatory, autonomic, and vascular processes. Anxiety disorders are more prevalent in areas with a high degree of urbanization. Access to recreational facilities, land-use mix, transportation systems, and urban planning and design are linked with overall cardiac health.

Nurses can corroborate these claims. Every day we see disease exacerbated by chronic stress, and chronic illness born of environmental factors. The field of epigenetics continues to shed light on these connections, demonstrating the ways our environment alters our health at the level of the chromosome, impacting which genes are expressed and which are silent.

Karen Silkwood and the doctor who looks to the water in the old saying are both upstream thinkers. They search for the root causes and determinants of disease, whether they are environmental or social. For public-policy makers, being an upstreamist means exploring environmental causes of disease in order to ameliorate challenges facing healthcare. For providers, it means focusing on preventive rather than reactive treatment, or focusing on the disease process much earlier on in its trajectory. For patients, it means sharing information you might not at first glance find relevant to your health.

Good providers and nurses consider general trends and sources of disease in addition to the biological evidence in front of them, but they need your communication to put the pieces together. If you live in hazardous conditions or you've experienced a significant life stressor (such as the death of a loved one, or a trauma), tell them. If you struggle with obesity, diabetes, or other variants of metabolic syndrome, ask them how your physical environment could be contributing to your disease. If you have asthma, discuss the places you spend the most time, and see if there might be a connection. Think about whether your friends or family members have struggled with what you're struggling with.

Being an upstreamist means learning to think beyond your symptoms and prompting your provider to do the same. Information you'd usually omit might end up being key to a diagnosis. If you don't take your environment into account, you might find relief — only to return to the places and circumstances that made you sick in the first place.

THREE:
APPOINT A TEAM

It's helpful to think about who you want on
your team — for the medical apocalypses
that might befall you over a lifetime, and to
help you keep the status quo the rest of the
time. Lacking this forethought means eventually having to navigate this foreign landscape as a lone citizen — without allegiances
or oracles on the inside. It means leaving it
up to chance that you'll find people who
are invested in you and will go the extra
mile to verse themselves in your case.
Anyone who's had a rude or incompetent
provider assigned to them or sat through an
appointment with one because it was the
only person with whom they could get an
appointment knows it's a gamble.

Gather a team that will look out for you
in sickness and in health, and do it while
the waters are calm. Don't try to secure
these positions urgently or reactively. It
takes time to build rapport with a provider,

familiarize yourself with resources, and choose the right person to be your advocate.

The following sections will walk you through finding an exceptional primary care provider and set you up for appointments that empower you rather than drain your will. They'll help you find providers and people in your peripheral vision who speak your language and tend to you with care and thoughtfulness within an imperfect, complicated system.

NORTH STAR: HOW TO CHOOSE A PRIMARY CARE PROVIDER

If I could yell one thing from the rooftops, it would be, *Get yourself a primary care provider!* I can't stress enough the importance of having one on your side as you navigate the world of medicine. Going through life without a PCP places more hurdles between you and the care you're trying to obtain. It's more of a hassle to go to a specialist, since many insurance carriers insist you have an appointment with your PCP and get a referral prior to going to, say, a pain specialist or a physical therapist. It also limits your options when you need that prescription from last year refilled or need advice for a sprain.

Whether it's a pediatrician for a kid, a

geriatrician for an older adult, a gynecologist for a woman, or a family medicine doctor at your neighborhood clinic — find one you have confidence in.

First, though, how *not* to choose one.

An American Household Converses About the Doctor

"It was my hands. It happened again."

"Jesus. Betty, you have to get this taken care of. That Dr. Patterson is not thorough. I swear, when we walked down Park Avenue, I could hear the quacking."

"I know. You've said that. But this doctor was nice. He was older, actually. He's from Rochester. He has two children. They're ten years apart."

— A CONVERSATION BETWEEN BETTY AND DON DRAPER. *MAD MEN,* SEASON 1, EPISODE 2.

Poor Betty. Here she is early on, tugging at our sympathies and fooling us into thinking she's a filler character — that is, until we watch her shield her eyes from the sun, cock a rifle, and go for the neighbors' pigeons with a Lucky Strike between her lips. In this scene, both distant and all too familiar, Betty does what many of us do when assessing a doctor. With a fifties sensibility, we look to their pedigree, their relatability, their likeness to *us*. If you read between the lines, what she's saying is:

He's got kids. A nice wife. A white picket fence and a degree from an Ivy. He's a man! So he must know what he's talking about when he says there's nothing physically wrong.

Betty's symptoms were declared a psychiatric problem, yet the nurse in me maintained they could have been from her thyroid, or neuropathy from too many cigarettes (she and Dr. Patterson were surely both smoking in his office), or early signs of her cancer. Might another doctor have gone further, done better? Spared her the long afternoons on a chaise longue in a psychiatrist's office when she could have been shooting pigeons to relieve stress? The show seems to imply that, yes, Patterson and some of the rest were lousy degenerates.

Don't choose providers just because they went to Yale, or because they look good on paper, or because your cousin's friend recommended them. Don't stick with one out of convenience, and definitely don't see someone who condescends to you or implies that a condition is imaginary. Finding the right primary care provider is a personal task, one that requires a little more vetting on your part (which we'll get to next).

For now, retire the old-school approach! And maybe even watch an episode of *The Bachelorette.* I hear it's a good reminder that there are always more fish in the sea.

How Are We Doing It Now?

The days of the family doctor — someone who knows your birthmarks and family history by heart and whose direct line is tucked away in your Rolodex — are essentially over. Today, the average adult sways like a pendulum between apathy and urgency when it comes to healthcare concerns, a custom that relies on outsourced care and doesn't necessitate having a relationship with any one person or place.

This is especially true up until middle age, a relatively quiet time for the majority, barring chronic illness and pregnancy. My friends in this age group (I've been one of them) tend to bounce from provider to provider: pediatrician, college health center, someone random at a walk-in clinic for a rapid strep test, Planned Parenthood for an IUD, a psychiatrist for Prozac.

So how *do* people decide who they see for their general care?

The answers are mixed. In the early 2000s, the answer was employers, ads, insurance networks, and recommendations from a friend or family member. Today it's those, plus some variation of "whoever I can get in to see that my insurance will cover."

Today, roughly 28 percent of men and 17 percent of women go without a PCP, a statistic that explains some patients' frustration with uncoordinated medical care. Among those who do have one, it's rare for them to see their PCP as a solid partner. The usual responses I get when asking how someone likes their doctor or nurse practitioner go something like:

"Mine is nice enough, but always in a rush."

"He's pretty awkward, but supposedly very good."

"I think I'd rather have a woman for this stuff. Should I see a woman?!"

"I want to see so-and-so, but I can't get in for four months."

"When I go to my [doctor's] office, a different person sees me every time. What do you mean, primary care provider?"

But some gush about their doctor or nurse practitioner, telling stories that make you think, *Damn, I deserve better!* So, onward and upward for the rest of us. It's a little much to compare finding a PCP to finding, say, a mate, but I insist that finding the right one is at least as important as choosing where to attend college, what company to work for, or where to go on vacation, tasks we greet with much more thought and enthusiasm.

Logistics of the Hunt

As you begin to hone your search for a PCP, consider the various types of providers who practice primary care. They include:

Family medicine physicians
Internists
General practitioners (GPs)
Ob-gyns (obstetrician-gynecologists) and gynecologists
Nurse practitioners (including family nurse practitioners, adult nurse practitioners, and women's health nurse practitioners)
Physician assistants
Pediatricians (for those up to twenty-one years old)

If you're coming in cold, the best way to commence the search is by asking providers and nurses you already know and like for a referral. This could be your therapist, your dentist, or a specialist you've seen at some point, or an immediate family member's provider (such as your child's or parent's provider). Next, ask friends and family directly. Finally, do a general search on the Internet. Apps like Zocdoc and Healthgrades can help you narrow down choices by reading reviews, but there always seem to be exceptional providers who don't show up on these sites because they keep a low profile, acquiring patients by word of mouth rather than advertising. This is all to say, begin with humans, then move to the web.

Once you've compiled a shortlist of people who might fit the bill, the next step is to find out if they're in network by calling their clinics and asking if the provider accepts your insurance. This is much easier than starting with an insurance network directory online and searching. Often these directories don't list all the provider's specialties — for example, a directory might not list that a family practice doctor also provides maternity care — and the information about whether they are accepting new patients is frequently out of date. Nurse practitioners employed by a physician practice may not be included in directories. Ultimately you'll get a narrower view of options using this platform.

Once you've found people who appear to be a good fit and accept your insurance, pare it down to two or three people based on the practice setting (discussed in the next section), their listed experience, and their location. You can then call the clinic or hospital where they practice, say you're looking to establish primary care, and ask if the person you're interested in offers meet and greets. Many — though not all — practices offer them, free of charge, for potential patients. You might only need to go to one of these to feel like you've found a good match, but there's no limit to how many providers you can interview. The meetings will also give you a chance to get a feel for the setting.

What to Look For
Next, what to look for once you're face-to-face, as well as information to help you evaluate a fit with your current PCP if you already have one.

While the right PCP might look very different from one person to the next, the best ones should possess certain traits. Take heart, by the way, in that this list was inspired by countless doctors and nurses I've witnessed model exceptional care throughout my career. They are out there, you just have to find them.

They Should Be Willing to Explain Their Thinking to You.

If you ask, they should be ready to walk you through how they came to a conclusion — or, better, they should offer on their own.

They Should Be Curious.

Curiosity is a worldview. It propels people toward presence and nimble thinking. Its absence is associated with burnout, ego, and a tendency toward conventionally accepted ideas rather than thinking critically and innovatively.

They Should Be Willing to Admit When Something Is Outside Their Wheelhouse.

Providers' not knowing something is more common than patients think, and admitting this is a crucial act of humility that can alter a course of care.

They Should Be Receptive Listeners.

Studies find that on average, physicians interrupt patients once every twelve seconds.[1] Pay attention to the way you engage in dialogue with a potential PCP and how they respond to what you say. If your provider consistently decides what is talked

78

about, where the conversation pivots, which questions are dismissed, and when a discussion of a particular item is over, there's a power imbalance. The *way* you talk might seem inconsequential compared to what you talk about, but if there's a power imbalance — even if the provider is perfectly delightful — exercising your agency will be an uphill battle. A battle you have to ultimately win, because when a provider exerts all the control in a conversation, it increases the risk that they will not get all they need to know from you and makes them more liable to take a wrong turn, getting both of you lost in the woods.

If you introduce a topic and the provider ignores it, or acknowledges it but quickly changes the subject, it means they've assigned a meaning to it that differs from yours. To find someone who listens is important, but to know you were *heard* is more complicated. Linguist Nancy Ainsworth-Vaughn writes, "Silence by one speaker makes time available for another speaker to talk. But silence itself cannot in any way demonstrate that the first speaker heard, understood, or cared about what was said. Talk can do that."

They Should Be Accessible.
Ask up front how accessible a potential PCP is:

If I needed to reach you in a health emergency, how would I go about doing that?

How much time, on average, are you able to spend face-to-face with a patient?

If I am admitted to a hospital where you have privileges, would you help co-ordinate my care?

What's the process if I need a prescription, or have a question for you but don't necessarily need to come in?

You're looking for potential hurdles here. In other words, what's between you and this person when you're out in the world and you need medical help? A receptionist? An operator line? An email? A text? A full-fledged appointment that must be scheduled and billed as such, even if the problem is minor? Be direct, and look for responses that answer your question rather than skirt it. Think of real predicaments you've been in before, when you've needed help and run into obstacles trying to get it. Answers about accessibility can vary greatly depending on the practice setting — we will get to the different models and what they offer patients in the section "Primary Care Models: The World Is Your Oyster" later.

They Should Speak Your Language.
The PCP you choose doesn't have to be someone you'd go get beers with, but they should speak your language and have a style and pace that feel comfortable to you.

If you're sensitive or introverted, look for someone you feel at ease around. If you want someone sharp and fresh, find a PCP who keeps up with the scientific literature. Maybe you want a provider with old-world charm, one who's seen it all from decades of experience, maybe this is what your parent would best respond to; or you might prefer a recently graduated MD with answers to the board exams still fresh in their minds. You can find a PCP with additional training in mental health or integrated medicine, if those are relevant for you. Aspects of your identity also factor in — culture, gender, sexual orientation, profession. These are part of your lived life, so you should be able to place them at the table with your PCP.

For practical reasons, your PCP needs to be convenient to you as well. This might mean a VA provider, or a preferred provider within your insurance network. For some, it means the provider has privileges at a certain hospital or is within a certain radius of their home.

Do Away with the Term "Bedside Manner"

I *never* want to hear the term "bedside manner" again! We use the term to explain why providers leave us in the dark, and to justify their bad behavior.

If someone can get through medical school, they can adopt basic conversational skills. A good provider is able to communicate with their patients. They will not always tell you what you want to hear, but they will never make you feel ashamed or belittled. Talking about weight, lifestyle choices, and reproductive health can be hard, and you'll likely ask questions whose answers seem plain as day to someone versed in medicine, but these circumstances never justify condescension. These qualities are not a matter of social grace or likability but of integrity and respect.

Poor bedside manner doesn't excuse not fulfilling basic responsibilities, especially when it comes to primary care. If you're facing a complicated surgery, you can consider letting someone less than charismatic cut you open or put you under, but a primary care provider who acts this way will fail you. The very nature of their role is to meet you where you are and invite ease and trust.

So if a PCP is aloof or unable to communicate with you effectively, try someone else. If a provider is crass or paternalistic, or you feel condescended to or judged in their presence — look elsewhere. Also watch out for the dismissive-with-a-guise-of-charm type. The research shows repeatedly that how a provider *makes you feel,* not merely the information they equip you with, can predict how you will interpret and manage your disease out in the world. Providers can leave you with a sense of control or no control depending on how they talk to you, even if they're perfectly polite.

Is It Better to See a Woman?
Over time I've gotten this question from female friends a lot, and I've asked it myself. When I'm trying to be evenhanded, the conclusion I come to is that, sure, you should see a woman provider if it makes you more comfortable. Why not? Some women don't want a pelvic exam from

someone who doesn't have a cervix, or feel safe discussing their reproductive health with a male. Do what makes you feel most comfortable — that's really what matters, I'd say.

Today I have a lot more to say on this subject. And I won't mince words: Women are, by many measures, superior doctors. Regardless of your sex, you should consider this when making healthcare decisions.

Here's what recent studies tell us. Female physicians are more likely to adhere to clinical guidelines,[2] counsel patients on preventive care,[3] and offer preventive screenings[4] than their male counterparts. According to research done in 2017 at the Harvard School of Public Health, patients who see a female internist have lower death rates and are less likely to be readmitted to the hospital within thirty days of discharge. Women doctors show greater empathy and are perceived as being better listeners, they are more communicative, they are more likely to practice evidence-based medicine, and they are less likely than their male counterparts to use humor to stop patients from talking.[5] Patients are also more satisfied with the care they receive from them.[6]

Women are better surgeons too.[7] Their patients have lower death rates, fewer complications, and lower readmissions to the hospital a month after their procedure, compared to the patients of male surgeons.

These trends have emerged in data that was collected as early as the nineties through today. The research has been challenged, but the findings are statistically significant across the board. The Harvard study is strong ammunition for quieting the critics: *The sample size was small!* some say. The study analyzed data from *1.6 million* hospital admissions. *The differences are negligible,* others conclude. "If we had a treatment that lowered mortality by 0.4 percentage points or half a percentage point [the same margin seen in the Harvard study], that is a treatment we would use widely. We would think of that as a clinically important treatment we want to use for our patients," Ashish Jha, professor of health policy at the Harvard School of Public Health, said in a *Washington Post* interview. In other words, the differences are *not* negligible.

Well then, something else must be influencing the data! others argue. But even after accounting for several relevant factors — such as the severity or type of patients' illness, the type of medical training, and the age or experience of the physicians — the findings remain largely the same. The last flimsy argument out there is that patients might just react better to female doctors, and that it has nothing to do with the actual care provided, to which I think, it's time to cut your losses.

If patients have better outcomes because they respond better to the care of female physicians, it means women doctors are providing patient-centered care, communicating more effectively, factoring in context, and empowering their patients. It means that the nature of communication and reciprocity between physician and patient is as or more salient to care outcomes than other components of the medical encounter.

These findings matter greatly because we are conditioned to think the opposite is true — that men are better doctors. Our culture tells us women are prone to emotions, fragile, not meant to wield a scalpel in an operating theater. They don't have the temperament to make life-and-death decisions. Men, on the other hand, are pragmatic and stoic, and have superior reasoning skills.

In a 2010 *Guardian* article, "Ten of the Best Good Doctors in Literature," all ten were men. Dr. Watson. Dr. Zhivago. The doctor who catches Lady Macbeth sleepwalking. The heroes of works like *Middle-*

march and *Arrowsmith.* In early films and novels, it was men who showed up with a black bag and saved little George before they won over the heroine at a fancy ball. Television and film have followed suit. We know the tropes: the young idealist who sets out to defy the system, the village hero who saves the boy from dysentery, the miserly doc who turns out to have a heart of gold, the lewd one who spanks a nurse here or there.

Even Doogie Howser appeared in living rooms across America before *ER* introduced Dr. Susan Lewis (who was a change from the 1974 screenplay on which the show was based — it centered on five white male doctors). It was the late nineties before women started to pop up with more regularity, and then Shonda Rhimes came along and changed all of it for good in 2005 with the premiere of *Grey's Anatomy.*

Meanwhile, women have, of course, been practicing medicine for centuries. Dr. Rebecca Lee Crumpler should be a household name. She earned her MD in 1864, the first black woman to do so in the United States. It goes without saying that women have made rich and remarkable contributions to the field of medicine dating back centuries. All along, the patriarchy insidiously and effectively made sure that as far as societal perception was concerned, the role of doctor and any social standing it afforded was reserved for men.

The cultural messages that shape our beliefs and mold our stereotypes often fly in the face of reality. Though representation of female physicians is perhaps more equal than in earlier years, they are still being paid less. All the while, many of them are doing a better job than their male counterparts.

So, see a woman doctor. Drive up demand so more enter the field. Consumer choice shapes healthcare, and when you see a female physician you're not only likely to get better care — you are voting for women.

Primary Care Models: The World Is Your Oyster

The diversity of primary care settings and setups leaves you with a few more things to factor into your decision before you choose a practitioner. Do you want more one-on-one time with your PCP? Unfettered access to them? Do you want a multidisciplinary team, or one that specializes in blending Eastern and Western medicine? Do you prefer to see a provider rooted in your local community, or one with a small practice who sees fewer patients and does almost everything themselves? Or do you move around so much that you'd like to streamline care with a national corporation with multiple sites?

Below are the three main types of primary care models, with their pros and cons elaborated on, followed by a list of settings and styles in which primary care is delivered today.

Traditional Practice ("Fee-for-Service")

How it works: This is the model most of us are familiar with. A patient chooses a PCP in their insurance network. The PCP bills the insurance company for services rendered, and the patient is responsible for paying the deductible and co-pays.

Pros: If you have a comprehensive insurance plan that provides free physicals and specific screenings, and covers or subsidizes medications, this model generally has the fewest out-of-pocket expenses.

Cons: In this model, providers at large clinics and hospitals (as opposed to private practice) may see upward of two thousand patients, meaning their time and attention are limited.

Approximate cost: Cost is highly dependent on insurance plan, but typical co-pays are $0 to $25 for well visits (physicals).

Direct Primary Care

How it works: This is a broad array of practice models that follow a retainer-based framework. The middle man is removed. No insurance party is involved, meaning patients pay providers directly. These practices offer routine care, preventive care, and care coordination, and some offer various types of specialty care (such as pediatrics or obstetrics), so they have less need to refer patients to specialists. They also often offer a discounted rate for services like imaging and lab tests.

Pros: These practices are small, capping out at five hundred to one thousand patients, and without the constraints of the traditional model providers have substantial time to dedicate to each case. This choice can be especially worthwhile for individuals with chronic pain, health anxiety, or long-term illness.

Cons: It's expensive, and still requires the patient to have a "wraparound" insurance plan to cover hospital stays, emergency care, and, ideally, some specialty care.

Approximate cost: The average cost to the patient begins at about $93 per month, before supplemental insurance.[8]

Concierge or Membership-Based Model

How it works: This is akin to joining a club. On top of any insurance plan, patients in these practices pay a membership fee to get direct access to a provider and additional "uncovered" services. For instance, the doctor might give out their cell number and text with patients.

Pros: This model offers unobstructed access to the provider and considerably more one-on-one attention, with added benefits like same-day appointments and house calls.

Cons: The cost is prohibitive for the

majority of folks, as it means paying fees (usually more expensive than direct primary care) on top of insurance premiums. And because there's a wide spectrum in cost and caliber, it takes a bit of research to find the best fit.

Approximate cost: The cost varies depending on practice. Boutique practices in New York can cost a family of four $80,000 per year, while other providers charge a flat fee of $1,500 to $2,000 annually, which the patient pays on top of insurance co-pays, deductibles, and any other fees.

Settings

Private practice: These clinics are typically out in the community and run by a single provider or a group of providers who work for themselves.

Community Health Center: These clinics provide care to medically underserved communities, and many take patients regardless of their ability to pay.

Hospital system: Large hospital consortiums such as Kaiser Permanente or the Mayo Clinic Health System house primary care divisions.

Teaching hospital: Teaching hospitals on the same campus as medical or nursing schools may house primary care offices or have affiliated primary care clinics offsite in neighboring communities. Massachusetts General Hospital and UCLA Medical Center are examples.

Styles

Traditional Western medicine: This is the prevalent care model in America. Healthcare professionals treat symptoms and diseases using drugs, lifestyle interventions, therapeutic interventions (for example, radiation), or surgery. You may also hear this style called allopathic medicine, conventional medicine, mainstream medicine, biomedicine, or orthodox medicine.

Functional medicine: If the body were a garden bed and its diseases weeds taking root and sprouting up, traditional medicine might look to specialists to eradicate the weeds and keep the vegetables growing. Functional medicine is more interested in the soil. Providers specializing in functional medicine employ a systems approach, meaning that rather than diagnosing and treating, they focus on identifying the root cause of diseases by closely examining patients' health history and environment.

Integrated/holistic medicine: Practices rooted in this type of care are where you'll find an emphasis on lifestyle, and an incorporation of Eastern practices such as acupuncture, herbalism, chiropractic care, and massage.

Osteopathic medicine: Have you ever seen a doctor with DO after their name instead of MD? This stands for "doctor of osteopathic medicine." Osteopathic medicine focuses on holistic, patient-centered care with a strong foundation in primary care. These providers have additional training in hands-on, manipulative medicine to alleviate pain and restore function to bodily systems.

With these models, more money does not necessarily translate to better care. While some primary care models allow for extended face time (and there are undoubtedly benefits to this), there are also superior practitioners working out in the community — the breadth of their experiences correlates directly to the diversity of cases they see, and allows them to come up with creative solutions to help people of all walks of life achieve optimum well-being. That said, Linda Laubenstein, who was among the first to discover and begin treating AIDS in the 1980s, operated from a private practice.

At the end of the day, primary care is really about the relationship between provider and patient — the setting is secondary.

OTHER MEDICAL PROFESSIONALS

It takes a village to stay on top of your healthcare needs. The following sections describe different types of care that often take a backseat to primary medical care, even though they're an essential part of the package.

Get a Mental Healthcare Provider Before You Need One

Mental and physical health are bound up with one another. Life stressors can cause and worsen disease, conditions and medications have psychological side effects, and having an illness can strike up its own mental health struggles. For these reasons, the medical world no longer considers mental health as accessory care, as it's integral to everything done to treat patients effectively.

One manifestation of this cultural shift is that today, an increasing number of primary care providers diagnose mental health conditions and prescribe medications for them. They're meeting a widespread need. Data collected from the National Prescription Audit shows that over half of psychiatric prescriptions written today are by general practitioners and primary care providers because, among other reasons, there's a shortage of specialists. Two thirds of the patients who receive psychiatric medications from their primary care provider say they go this route because they're unable to access psychiatric treatment.[9]

While addressing mental health needs in primary care is a viable route, and a sound one to use if you need immediate help, most mental health conditions require specialty care and dedicated attention beyond what is available in these settings. Something many people don't realize until they're in dire straits and can't wait, however, is that when you don't have care established with a mental health clinician, options for timely help are limited, and it may take several months for an intake appointment. Getting an intake appointment? It's no small feat, and it's often the last thing one has the patience and motivation for when feeling badly.

If you suffer a traumatic event or an unexpected loss or if you've become a servant to anxiety or sadness for unknown reasons, making the decision to get professional help can be a difficult task in its own right. It seems like summoning the grit this decision demands should be the hardest part of the process. Unfortunately, it's just the beginning of a series of hurdles. Next you have to browse a list of strangers online, trying to choose someone you could potentially cry in front of from a sea of headshots and vague bios. Then you have to make cold calls and emails to see if these providers are accepting new patients. You also have to tackle the insurance piece and, if you need one, get a referral.

Finding a clinician who accepts new patients can prove especially challenging, because there aren't enough psychiatric providers to meet patient demand. This can be true of counselors and therapists, but it's even more so for clinicians with the ability to prescribe (psychiatrists and psychiatric nurse practitioners). The average wait time before you can be seen for a first appointment is thirty days, or sixty during busier periods like the winter holidays and back-to-school.

This challenging process, made more difficult by the system's red tape, confuses and frustrates patients, as there are few actionable things one can do to expedite care when they really can't wait sixty days to feel better. The current reality is that unless an individual is in imminent danger, they are not a fit for an inpatient setting, and their options for help in the immediate sense are limited. They include waiting until the light of day, getting an intake appointment, or going to your PCP for a prescription and what may be a crude diagnosis in the interim.

If help cannot wait, primary care is a good bridge of support while you establish mental healthcare, and I advocate going to a PCP for this purpose. There's yet another option, however, that might help you circumvent the entire process with a little foresight.

Last autumn, on a walk, someone close to me and very insightful — who has a way of seeing the obvious where I cannot — explained why she established care with a therapist before she really needed one, and was continually glad she had. Hearing this was an epiphany. So immersed in the field I sometimes can't see the forest for the trees, I realized what an important notion it is, and how often patients and providers don't think in these terms. This preventative measure, taken when things are status quo, not only affords you the time to choose a good fit, but it also puts infrastructure in place to support you when the unexpected happens.

Getting a therapist or other psychiatric provider before you need one doesn't mean you need to see them weekly, but it does mean selecting a provider and maintaining a relationship with them. An invaluable resource when you need to be seen immediately, it also allows you to leisurely choose someone whose style and practice suit your needs, as you would a primary care provider.

Keep in mind that finding a mental health-care provider can be a lengthy and arduous task — and my recommendation may place more strain on a system already stretched thin. But putting in the effort up front to find someone who's the right amount of gentle, funny, wise, or challenging is well worth it. Contact and set up intake appointments with two to three professionals before deciding on one to maintain care with. Often, these "see-if-we're-a-fit" appointments come at a nominal fee, or are complimentary, when the professional is a therapist or LCSW (licensed clinical social worker). You will need to determine the cost of more formal intake appointments with psychiatrists or psychiatric NPs on a case-by-case basis. It will come down to your insurance coverage and whether the provider works for a large system or in a private practice.

If you are interested in seeking care with an emphasis on talk therapy, then counselors, therapists, and psychologists are a good fit. If you have a family or personal history of more complex mental health issues (major depression unresponsive to treatment, bipolar-type disorders, eating disorders, or generalized anxiety, for example), it could benefit you to work with a psychiatrist or psychiatric NP who specializes in these disorders and can use pharmacological intervention in addition to therapy.

Getting in to see a new mental health provider is the most difficult during fall and winter (between September and January). Around the holidays, travel and time off commence, inclement weather can set schedules back, and strained family relations, patterns of grief, and the stress of holiday activities make providers even busier. Calling at this time usually means the intake appointment will be two to three months out — which may work fine for you.

Some progressive cities, like Portland and Los Angeles, offer community-funded walk-in clinics that help those without insurance get psychiatric medication, or provide them with someone to seek guidance from in an escalating situation. If you need to renew a prescription you've had previously or get on a medication while you wait to be seen by your regular provider, you can use the Substance Abuse and Mental Health Services Administration (http://findtreatment.samhsa.gov) to look up these clinics in your area online, or call for advice 24/7.

Eyes and Teeth: The Medical Silos
Dental and vision care operate under distinct systems in both medical and economic models. It's illogical and antiquated, but somehow they are silos, assigned unequal status in the eyes of the medical establishment and insurance programs. Receiving an immunization for whooping cough or seeing a specialist for athlete's foot is likely to be covered by insurance, but if you need

glasses to see, that's another story! Medicaid programs acknowledge the need for dental care only in children and pregnant women.

Many patients now triage the needs of their eyes and teeth, either because these appointments are not covered and thus prohibitively expensive or because patients are, understandably, taking the medical system's lead. If the world of medicine annexes vision and dental, carving out only minimal space to discuss them in medical contexts, they must not be that important. This message is in fact so misleading!

Don't treat them as silos. They are partitioned because of policy and because systems are set in their ways, and not because of their relevance to overall physical health. Dental and vision history needs to be part of your medical history, and clinicians working on your eyes and teeth should be in communication with your primary care provider about any major diagnoses or planned procedures. Here are the basics on taking care of these two amazing sensory organs.

Vision

I have truly terrible vision. If I'd been born before the first bifocals were invented in the thirteenth century, I'd have been sentenced to a life of navigating one big indistinguishable blur. Despite this profound dependence on modern optometry, I, like many, take it for granted.

Until a few years ago, I was guilty of not always taking the best care of my eyes. But one day, I was sitting in a dark exam room at a clinic named something cute, like Blink, irritated about the exorbitant fee I had to pay just to get my prescription for contacts renewed. The optometrist started oohing and aahing at something she found while running a blinding strand of light across my retina.

Apparently I had a rare eyeball anomaly that put me at risk for retinal detachment. Dilated — and jarred by this new information that I could go blind in my left eye at any moment (in fact, she made it seem like a true miracle that it hadn't happened yet) — I was caught off guard. We went on to have a discussion about my risk of glaucoma based on my medical history, as well as my options and what I could do to stave it off. The whole experience mirrored a medical appointment, though I'd gone in treating it as nonchalantly as if it were a dress fitting.

Contacts and glasses are outlandishly expensive, and you're trapped into having an eye exam every time you need them replaced or the prescription renewed, which is usually annually. Most insurance plans either don't offer vision coverage or offer it only as an expensive add-on. So it's not a surprise that it's often the first thing you eliminate when you're sorting out a health-care budget.

Yet eye exams are about more than being able to see leaves and letters as crisply as possible. They assess for the presence and risk of major eye conditions, such as glaucoma, macular degeneration, and vascular damage from conditions like diabetes. And who's to say what will come of our collective endless stare into the blue light of our computers and phones, the ramifications of which we don't yet understand. Modern eyes are strained, and they're beginning to let us know! Staying on top of eye conditions in their early stages will help you maintain eye health for as long as possible, so you can keep reading books and admiring the flowers into old age.

Lastly, contact lenses are not the easiest thing in the world, and they come with their own set of hazards, like corneal abrasions and infections. Anyone who's suffered from these can attest to their awful discomfort, but how long you have to wait for the blessed anesthetizing drops to soothe the pain will depend on if you have an optome-trist to call.

Below are ways to maximize the resources available to the public for eye care.

Types of eye specialists

Here are the different types of eye special-ists, so you know who to go to for what:

Ophthalmologist: A physician who can diagnose and treat complicated eye problems, such as glaucoma, and per-form surgery.

Optometrist: A doctor of optometry, who carries out basic eye exams and writes prescriptions for lenses.

Optician: A trained professional who sells glasses and fills prescriptions.

Buying contacts online

Once you've had a vision exam and gotten a prescription, providers will usually give you the option of purchasing contacts or glasses directly in the clinic. But it's often less expensive to go online. It's a good idea to at least have a sense of what your brand costs online to see if pricing in the clinic is comparable.

Using senior discounts

EyeCare America, a program of the American Academy of Ophthalmology, helps eligible seniors obtain free or discounted vision care. The AARP, the American Automobile Association (AAA), and the Department of Veteran Affairs (VA) also offer great discounts for seniors on eye care.

Are routine visits worth paying for out of pocket? Yes. The approximate cost of an eye exam is $100, and it's well worth it, especially if you use corrective lenses. Extreme nearsightedness ups your chances of having retinal problems, so if you're blind like me don't get too behind on your appointments!

Teeth

If the eyes are the window to the soul, the gums are the window to systemic health. I heard a statistic on the radio the other day that dogs live two to five years longer if you floss their teeth a few times a month. I'm not sure my retriever or I have it in us for that battle, but for some reason it convinced me — more than any lecture from a dentist or my dad (a former navy dental tech) — that we wildly underestimate the importance of oral health.

When you're sitting open-mouthed in the

dental chair while a hygienist glides an instrument along your gumline, calling out "2's," "3's," and "4's" in rapid succession, they're testing for inflammation. They've adopted this practice because the literature has demonstrated a clear link between gum inflammation and heart inflammation. Evidence suggests that oral bacteria could play a key role in creating the fatty deposits that clog arteries, contributing to strokes and cardiovascular disease.[10] There seems to be a clear link to fetal development as well, as the *Iranian Journal of Reproductive Medicine* came out with a study in recent years demonstrating that for pregnant women, periodontitis (a serious gum infection) can cause premature birth and low birth weight.[11]

Medical professionals have always understood the importance of dental health, but only in recent years has the dentist been rightfully recognized as an essential component of your primary healthcare team, rather than an adjunct specialist. Patients should follow suit.

To make sure you get the most out of every cleaning, be sure to discuss any major health conditions with your dental team, especially if you are pregnant or have a history of cardiovascular issues. Relay this information face-to-face, and before latexed hands are in your mouth! If the exam reveals high levels of inflammation or your dentist has other specific concerns, get a copy of your records, discuss them with your PCP, and have them added to your medical chart. Consult your PCP about any major dental work you're having done (particularly root canals), especially if you have heart disease. In rare cases intense dental procedures may introduce bacteria to the bloodstream which can inflame the heart's lining, so your PCP may want you on protective antibiotics before the dental procedure.

Can't afford the dentist?
Try a dental school! Dental school clinics can save you as much as 75 percent on care, and they often offer free screenings. Another option for underserved communities, and for older adults who have difficulty traveling, is mobile dental clinics. These exist in several but not all states, so finding one requires a quick Internet search on the front end.

Befriend Your Pharmacist
Sometimes I feel a twinge of guilt when I check the "Decline pharmacist counseling"

box on the drugstore checkout pad. It's most often an act of stubbornness. Until I became a nurse, my interactions with pharmacists were cursory and often came with a dose of irritation born of waiting — on a doctor's sign-off, for an insurance company's approval, or in a long line of people coughing.

Then I learned there's *so* much more to a pharmacy than I appreciated. I got my schooling on the subject in 2015, while making home visits to newly arrived refugees to help navigate their medical issues. I'd arrive as part of a team: a medical student, a nursing student, and, if we were lucky and schedules aligned, a pharmacy student.

As patients, we tend to think of pharmacists as working in community retail settings, doling out our pain meds and antibiotics. But they're actually an integral part of the medical model, and a good portion hold positions in hospitals. In writing this section, I Googled "How many drugs exist in the US market?" The first link was a Quora site on which the first comment was, "Are you serious?" I laughed to myself only because it illustrates the infinite number of prescription drugs we take. The answer: *10,562.*

Pharmacists are akin to drug encyclopedias. They're trained to know the details of absorption, indications, side effects, and potentially life-threatening interactions of the medications we ingest. When a patient or provider can't find an answer, pharmacists are the savviest and most efficient at searching the scientific literature. We nurses and doctors rely heavily on their expertise so we can focus on the person and diagnosis in front of us.

The chain of accountability, or checks and balances, keeps patients safe in the hospital. (See page 373 for an exact breakdown of a hospital order and all the hands it must pass through before getting to the patient.) Without pharmacists, this chain would unravel quickly. They're the veritable gatekeepers of the hospital, guarding a vault of medications that they won't dole out unless they're safe and indicated for patients.

Have you ever wondered if a nagging headache is related to your heart medication? If you need to worry about a painkiller crossing the placenta? If combining Tylenol with another of your medications could be dangerous? Pharmacists possess a rich assortment of facts that extend beyond the instructions on a pill bottle. In some cases, their knowledge might even save you a trip or call to the doctor. Befriend them. Get to know one at the retail store you get prescriptions from so you have a consistent person you can go to with questions about prescription (Rx) and over-the-counter (OTC) medications. When you're asked to step to the next window so a pharmacist can counsel you, take advantage of their expertise and ask whatever you want. If you're in the hospital and have concerns about medications you're receiving and want to talk to a pharmacist directly, ask for one to visit your room.

Alternative Care

Alternative medicine, an umbrella term for complementary alternative medicine, Eastern medicine, and integrative care, is a significant source of interest and healing for lots of patients. If you're wanting to learn more about options that might complement your traditional care, the government's National Center for Complementary and Integrative Health is the place to start investigating.

If you *are* going to seek integrative medicine, you have to integrate it. It's a resource to help treat the root causes and side effects of illness, but it should be used in conjunction with the rest of your healthcare. It's your responsibility to have your integrative and traditional providers communicate with each other, unless both are housed in the same practice (a larger discussion on your role in care coordination can be found on page 276).

To integrate the care, ask alternative practitioners up front if they're willing to be part of a team and work with your conventional providers. Also ask this of your Western medical team, especially your PCP. My general rule of thumb is to be wary of anyone who rejects this collaboration, or who implies they should be your sole source of care.

CHOOSING AN ADVOCATE: DON'T GO TO APPOINTMENTS ALONE

For one of the patient interviews for this book, I met a woman in her late eighties. We'll call her Martha. Martha is one of those people who intuits how to be a patient, and she was doing it well long before I was born. We spent a sunny fall afternoon having coffees in her backyard, and she educated me. Among her stories was one that led to this section.

Martha is, among other things, a bioethicist with an incredible breadth of knowledge about the healthcare system and medical ethics. Decades ago she testified as an expert witness on why women who have received a diagnosis of breast cancer should be given written information about their disease and treatment options to take when they leave the office.

Today, written information is given out as a matter of course at most clinics and hospitals. (Just the other day, I walked out with a thick pile of paper explaining a sinus infection!) But back in the seventies and eighties, this wasn't the case. Ultimately, Martha's testimony — and the work in recent decades of others devoted to patient rights — put laws in place that require that patients get written information before they walk out the door, especially when they've received a new, long-term diagnosis.

Getting the news that you have a malignancy or a chronic illness is a traumatic moment for the average person. More than emotional, it puts the body in an activated fight-or-flight state, the blood diverted away from the parts of our brain we need to take in new information. To make decisions about new information, you have to learn new things, and this requires a calm state. If you have written information, you can take it in once you've had time to process the new reality.

Martha's story and the medical system's acknowledgment of this innate human response are relevant to situations across the healthcare continuum, not just receiving a diagnosis (though this is where it's most salient). The same fight-or-flight reaction and compromised ability to take in new information is also at play if you're nervous before a routine appointment, or when you're at the hospital and getting information about your condition.

More broadly, people in modern society tend to be chronically stressed, repeating the stress response over and over so many times throughout the day that it's more like a through line than a cycle. This means you could have a fight-or-flight reaction at any point of any interaction with medicine, depending on how your day, year, or life is going.

Because of this, and the current fractured state of the medical system, I think you should never enter the world of modern medicine alone, if you can help it. Whether it's for major surgery or your annual physical, routine or emergency or follow-up.

I know — it's extreme in nature, inconvenient in practice, and perhaps even uncomfortable in theory for the lone wolves of the world, but the times demand it.

Two is better than one at a medical encounter. Being a patient requires multitasking, but we're only human, with only so many arms and so much capacity to listen — especially when we're stressed. When more information is being exchanged than one person can handle (as happens in most medical encounters), an extra brain is good. When medical error is so common in hospitals, an extra set of eyes and ears is good. And, in the event it's delivered, it's often easier to absorb difficult news with someone who supports you.

Think of sleepaway camp, and the protection system used in lakes during all the splashing and merrymaking. Drowning is always a risk, especially when it comes to little swimmers who outnumber the two or three teen lifeguards. So camps implement a buddy system and assign each camper a "protector" who's always looking out for them, placing an additional set of eyes on each swimmer as they drift in and out of the counselor's field of vision. The lifeguards are still ultimately responsible for everyone, and they might be the only ones who know CPR, but the buddies create another layer of safety. Water clarity can impact lifeguards' ability to see from an elevated vantage point. Wind may impact their ability to hear.

A poor swimmer may disproportionately consume their attention. Buddies compensate for lifeguards' blind spots and, in doing so, maintain a lifeline that's saved many a child from drowning.

Hospitals are where our minds usually go when we hear the word "advocate." In hospitals, when patients are preoccupied or sick, their ability to advocate for themselves is compromised. When providers are stretched thin and overburdened with responsibility, channels of communication break down and things fall through the cracks. So an advocate is particularly vital here, where consequences can be grave and immediate. But they're also valuable at regular appointments, where patients may be processing difficult news or forget to attend to all the bullet points on their list because they're fatigued or distracted. In these spaces, an advocate can step in and significantly impact health outcomes.

It serves every patient — every person — to have a healthcare advocate. And it's too important a matter for you to handle it on an ad hoc basis, grabbing a different friend or family member willing to accompany you to every appointment.

Who Should It Be?

When you're choosing an advocate, start by thinking of someone in your life who is dependable, conscientious, loyal, and sharp. You could ask a friend who's a nurse, physician, or other type of healthcare professional, as their knowledge and experience make for excellent advocacy. It doesn't have to be someone in your immediate tribe. It could be your partner, parent, child, or longtime friend, but it could also be your neighbor or librarian, as long as you have enough rapport with them to make this request.

I see lots of patients (especially elderly people, people with insecure housing, and people with severe mental health issues) who lack a support network and don't even have visitors in the hospital, let alone people to step up and help them. So in a sense, making a paradigm shift so that everyone has access to an advocate is a social justice issue: When people begin to use health advocates more often, we will begin to normalize the practice and integrate it into the healthcare world. This role will become expected, appreciated, and thought of as standard for everyone, and resources will be allotted to make that happen. A dream of mine, anyway . . .

How Can They Help?

If you've ever been to an appointment with a friend, or had a partner or family member with you in the hospital, you've probably seen that people who accompany you to medical encounters naturally assume the advocate role. The information below can give them additional ways to help — and a well-earned title for all their work!

At Appointments

If you have a chief complaint and you're preparing for an appointment to discuss it, you can share your elevator story with your advocate (see "Creating an Elevator Complaint," page 202). You can practice on them before going to the appointment, if that's helpful, or give them a copy so they can make sure you stick to the script the day of. If the appointment is routine and your preparation entails listing your questions and topics you need to cover, your advocate can serve a similar role. It's easy to forget something during the rushed, nervous energy of an appointment, so have someone provide back up.

Below is an excellent list of questions for people advocating for patients at medical appointments. (The AARP made it for people advocating for their parents, but you can adapt the questions for a patient of any age.) You can give them to your advocate to mull over before the appointment or reference during it.

Diagnoses

What illness or condition do/could they have?
How is the condition or illness diagnosed?
What are the treatment options?
What is the most effective treatment?
What are the causes of this condition or illness?
What is likely to happen with and without treatment?
Are there common complications associated with this illness or condition?

Medications

What is the name of the medicine you are prescribing?
What is its benefit?
Is a generic drug available?
What are the risks and side effects?
How often should they take the drug?
How long should they take the drug?
What foods, other medicines, or activities should they avoid while taking this drug?

Could this medicine interact with any
medications they are currently taking?

Tests

Are tests necessary?
What will they show?
What preparation is needed?
When will we get the results?
What do the test results mean?

Surgeries

Why does my loved one need surgery?
How is the surgery performed?
Where will the surgery be performed?
Are there alternatives to surgery?
What risks are associated with this opera-
tion?
What kind of anesthesia will be used?
What is the average recovery time?
How much experience do you have per-
forming this type of surgery?

Costs

What costs can we expect?
Will insurance cover this test or treatment?
What can we do to reduce costs?

Written instructions

Do you have any written information that
we can take home?

Follow-up care

Is a follow-up visit necessary? If so, when
should we follow up?
If we think of questions later, how can we
contact you?

In the Hospital
When a patient is hospitalized, an advocate
is something of a watchdog. They can also
orchestrate coordination and communication between all the parties that become
involved with care. An advocate can:

Educate themselves about the signs and
symptoms of common complications
and keep an eye out for them
Make sure they're present for rounds if
the patient is sleeping or unable to
participate
Call the rapid-response team if they have
a concern and the professionals on the
floor have not intervened (see "When
No One Is Listening")
Call a meeting if they feel that different

121

specialists or departments aren't talking to one another

Keep an eye on vital signs for anything that indicates a problem (see the section "Keep an Eye on Vitals," page 398, to learn exactly how)

There are countless ways an advocate can look out for someone in the hospital. You can find other specifics throughout the book, especially in "When You're Not the Patient: Family Members, Partners, and Friends." Ultimately, any suggestion or idea in this book that a patient needs help implementing or navigating can be the work of an advocate.

Special Circumstances

When things are really serious and sudden, especially around a hospitalization or an unexpected trauma, the role of advocate can be too much to place on a friend or family member who's attempting to cope. The learning curve required here can be too steep. In this case, it can be helpful to designate as advocate a person *outside* the immediate picture. This person can even be out-of-state — as long as they have a computer, a phone, and a level head, they don't necessarily need to be there physically.

If there's an emergency and a friend or cousin asks if there's anything they can do — this is something they can do. Just make sure you pick someone who has the strengths, and the time, to dedicate to the role. I also don't recommend having multiple advocates for the same situation; try to keep it centralized with one person. Everyone can be there and help and support the patient, but you know the old adage — too many cooks in the kitchen . . .

Four:
Gather Provisions

Do you know off the top of your head the dosage of all the medications you take? Whether your paternal grandfather had liver disease? What year you got that immunization as a baby? If someone found you unconscious would they be able to find out whether you have a medical condition? The following sections will identify the provisions you'll need when you enter the world of modern medicine — from a dossier of your medical records, to a family tree, to medical identifiers listed in your phone.

CREATE A MEDICAL DOSSIER

The Healthbook
Invest in a notebook dedicated just to being a patient. You can use it to take notes during appointments, write down questions you'd like to ask your provider as you think of them, and draw out a family tree com-

plete with medical history. It also comes in handy in hospital settings, when you need to keep track of the chaos (see page 368 on how to use it there). Whether you take pen to paper or prefer the smartphone equivalent, create a centralized place for jotting down and storing important information. Including or linking to a calendar is a great idea as well!

I also recommend that patients and their friends keep a directory of names and contact information for all their providers, their pharmacy location and phone number, their advocate contact information, and clinics they go to for any specialty care. In this sense, your healthbook can function as a Rolodex as well.

Your Medical Records
No single person presides over your medical information. Providers access it when necessary and maintain its security, but no one ensures that it's used to its fullest potential. But from now on, you are going to do this.

The backbone of this provisions list is a copy of your medical records — something many patients don't possess, and don't know they can request. This dossier should grow with you over time, and it's enormously helpful to have it accessible.

Presiding over this information ensures that your care is coordinated and based off a central source of complete, up-to-date information. It allows your full medical history to follow you to every specialist appointment. It prevents duplicate testing. It often holds clues to diagnoses that can only be discovered in context — context providers often don't have the time to go digging for on their own.

Having a compilation of your medical records and familiarizing yourself with its contents increases your chances of accurate diagnosis and helps prevent medical error. When you're privy to the same information as your providers, you can better advocate for yourself. There are times the simple act of carrying the information with you into an appointment and being sure parts of it are read, knowing that you and your provider have your eyes on the same information and can process it together, can change the outcome. Ultimately, the record is your best assurance that both you and your team are getting a whole and accurate story.

Acquiring this will also make your life easier. You won't need to call the clinic, explain why you need the information you do, and get shuffled through an automated system for every quick bit of information. *When was that last vaccine? Did I end up getting that screening done, and what year was it? When did those symptoms start? Did the hospital actually spend four hours on the surgery I'm about to pay my insurance for?*

More protected and less accessible than their paper ancestors, modern medical records can be a challenge to obtain. Individual patient records used to live in weathered manila file folders. Requesting a fax or a copy was a fairly uncomplicated exchange: ask, xerox, done. With the shift to electronic medical records, though, your history, test results, and hospitalization information live in the cloud. While they may have changed in form, the system that presides over their use has not. The Health Insurance Portability and Accountability Act (HIPAA) created a padlocked system, built to cloister and safeguard sensitive and personal details and keep them out of the wrong hands. This is, of course, *very* important. There is a reason HIPAA rules the medical world. But because of it, no one encourages shuffling around medical files. Your records are available to you only if you ask. But they're *your* records — obtaining them is a federal right that trumps state variations or office policies regarding the request process. It still might be a royal pain to collect them, though, so treat yourself to something nice once you've succeeded.

Below, you'll find a guide to obtaining and compiling your records that should help you trounce any stumbling blocks or professional mules that hassle you along the way.

Collecting Your Medical Records

If you go to a large hospital or clinic, call the operator and ask to be connected with the health information management (HIM) department. If you work with a smaller office, call and explain that you'd like to access your records and ask to be directed to the right person.

Once connected, ask to sign a patient access request form or similarly titled document. On the form, you'll indicate which portion of your records you're requesting. Check all the boxes if you're starting from scratch. This may raise a few brows, as the documents can be a hundred-plus pages, but that's okay. You can typically sign this form online and return it via email.

Things to Keep in Mind:

You will have to prove you are indeed yourself, either via photo identification upon pickup or with your social security number.

HIPAA does not allow the release of very specific portions of medical information — such as psychotherapy notes.

Decide what format you'd like to receive the file in. You can typically choose between CD, flash drive, and secure email. Talk with the HIM or record coordinator about your options when you call.

There may be a fee associated with the labor for obtaining the records. If you request the information electronically, the cost is legally bound to be $6.50 or less, so do not overpay. Federal regulations are actually working to make these records more accessible to patients and to reduce their cost, so as time goes on, you will be more likely to find that there's no fee.

Medical organizations can take up to thirty days to fulfill the request and deliver your records, but usually it won't take this long. I'd estimate ten days or so.

You'll need to repeat these steps for each clinic or hospital you've been seen at. It's an arduous process, but it could be rather sweet to call your old pediatrician's office to say hello and tell them about all you've accomplished since kindergarten!

See What You're Made Of

Did your uncle eat fried chicken and drink sweet tea and still live to be ninety-seven?

What was the type of breast cancer your mother's sister had? Was it pre- or postmenopausal? Was she tested to see if it was hereditary?

Family trees may sound like the stuff of grade-school show-and-tell, but you should create one and file it with other important health documents. It's a useful tool to determine what types of screenings you should have done, at what age, and with what frequency. It also tunes your provider in to your personal risk profile so you can tailor prevention plans (where possible) for inheritable and preventable conditions, like diabetes or heart disease. With a solid, complete family health history to refer to, rather than facts tossed out at random during appointments, your provider can better help you determine a plan.

If anyone in your family has had one of these, be sure to tell your provider up front, in the early days of your routine care:

Breast, ovarian, or uterine cancer
Colon, pancreatic, or prostate cancer
Thyroid disorder
Heart disease

Type 2 diabetes
Stroke
Melanoma
Osteoporosis

How to Create a Family History Tree

You can create your own chart (ideally in your healthbook) and share it with your provider, or you can enter the information into the surgeon general's My Family Health Portrait tool (http://familyhistory.hhs .gov).

Begin by writing down the names of all your blood relatives, beginning with parents, siblings, and children, then moving on to grandparents, aunts, uncles, nieces, nephews, and half siblings. Ask family members about any chronic diseases and conditions they have had (such as heart disease, diabetes, stroke, high blood pressure, cancer, asthma, dementia, and multiple sclerosis) and at what age they were diagnosed. Find out the age and cause of death for any relatives no longer around.

Also consider your family's heritage and ancestry. Were they Vikings? Ashkenazi Jews? Refugees whose origins are unknown? If you don't know, that's important to note too.

At each turn, seek nuance and detail. If you're able, find out specifics about the manifestation of any disease and its progress. Did it respond to treatment? Did the family member attempt lifestyle changes (in the case of diabetes or heart disease)? Did cancer recur or go into remission? Find out the exact diagnosis, if possible — for example, oat-cell carcinoma, as opposed to the more general lung cancer; ductal carcinoma, as opposed to breast cancer. Was dementia vascular? Lewy body? Not all types are Alzheimer's. Providers don't expect the majority of patients to go to this length to collect detail, but the information will result in more precise care.

Friends in the Digital Age

I am not a proponent of screens standing between people. Talking to a healthcare provider these days can resemble checking in for a flight! But I've met my waterloo with this one — technology isn't going anywhere. (I also think of those days I went to work with my mom as a little girl, playing in a library of medical charts flagged with colored tabs and alphabetized by last name, and it seems prehistoric.) Even I can admire the benefits of the massive overhaul of paper medical records.

Two of these benefits that can help you as a patient are Care Everywhere and

MyChart.*

Care Everywhere is a feature of electronic medical records that swiftly and securely exchanges medical information between healthcare professionals. Your chart once had to be requested, thumbed through, signed off on, and faxed, but providers can now access it simply by clicking "outside record" and querying for the information they need, getting it in a matter of seconds.

This is lovely, because it means that rather than being tied to a place, medical information is tied to a *patient* moving through the world. You don't have to stress as much about exact dates and places, or results you can't recall; you can simply ask your provider to look them up. Having this information at their fingertips helps both providers and patients. And if your security alarm is going off, just remember that only the healthcare professionals *directly working with you during the visit* have access to the information. Care Everywhere does not replace the need to have your own copy of your

* Note, the material in this section is based off of Epic, a commonly used electronic medical records system in US hospitals. Semiequivalents exist with other EMR programs. Inquire with your clinic or hospital which EMR system is used.

medical records (see "Create a Medical Dossier," page 124), as the full record grants shared access to broad strokes of information like patterns, family history, and chronology, but Care Everywhere can get quick answers on the exact date of a procedure or result of a test in real time.

You're more likely to have heard of My-Chart, as you've probably been encouraged to sign up for this online portal. It has an online dashboard allowing you to communicate with your provider, request appointments, refill prescriptions, and access portions of your medical records. Though I'm a bit more skeptical about this one — it can feel like yet another way to economize on healthcare delivery and minimize the need for human interaction — there are definite benefits, and I recommend signing up. Outside of the main tools and features available, here are some less obvious ways to use the portal to your advantage:

Loop in your advocate (see the section "Choosing an Advocate," page 112). MyChart offers a way to give another person access to the details they need to best support you. Using the proxy access form (which can be downloaded from MyChart or requested from clinic staff), you can designate another adult or adults you'd like to have access to your account. This will allow them to bypass bureaucratic formalities when they are trying to get information about your condition. People to consider granting access to include:

 Spouses or partners
 Children (especially as you age)
 Parents
 Friends
 Your health advocate

Ask your provider questions. If you have a specific, nonemergency question or request — one that does not require a conversation but simply a yes-or-no answer — you can use MyChart to message your provider. Expect to hear back in one to three days.

Prepare for appointments. If you have an appointment coming up, you can use MyChart to message your provider and brief them on why you're coming in. Don't be long-winded, but relay the general points to prep for the conversation and ensure that you will talk about everything you wanted. It's a useful way to maximize your face-to-face time. You can also use the feature if you have an appointment coming up to discuss a specific test result: check-in ahead and make sure it's been received before you trek to the office!

YOUR SMARTPHONE AS A MEDICAL DEVICE

The advent of smartphones has affected most facets of the healthcare system — for patients as well as clinicians. Voice memos replaced Dictaphones, the Internet now houses extensive libraries of medical literature, pharmacies send text alerts about prescription refills, and apps allow patients to do everything from accessing their records to cataloging their medications to finding the best specialists in their vicinity.

Virtual Toolbox

Your phone itself contains a number of simple features — ones you're already familiar with — that you can use both in and out of appointments to make you a safer, more informed patient. These include health app, photos, voice recordings, and notes.

How to Set Up Your Medical ID

To make your important health information accessible in the event of an emergency, set up your Medical ID in the Health app on your iPhone or with the built-in Android feature. Stop now (yes, literally, now!), pull out your phone, and take a few moments to set it up. In a mad rush to put you back together in an emergency, responders and medical teams have to quickly determine your identity, medical history, allergies, medications, and emergency contact. The Medical ID — which can be accessed without unlocking your phone — can save them valuable time.

How to Use Photos

There are countless types, brands, and styles of medical devices. You should have full information on hand about the ones you use so you can answer any questions about them that come up at an appointment, with a pharmacist, or in a hospital setting. I recommend taking photos of your medical equipment that you can easily access at appointments. That way, you can verify that you and the nurse, provider, or physical therapist are talking about the same thing. Instead of trying to describe an obscure piece of equipment that your previous specialist had you using, you've got the real thing in front of your and the provider's eyes. On many occasions I've had patients arrive on the hospital unit, with their partners scrambling around trying to find the patient's inhaler, brace, or CPAP nozzle. It's easy to replace these in hospitals, but it helps if we know exactly what make and model we're dealing with instead of a description of a thingamabob.

The antidote to confusion can be as simple as a few shots on your phone, stored in an accessible folder. Snap images of any equipment you use, and be sure the brand is visible. Here are a few examples of devices you should get pictures of:

Insulin pumps
Inhalers
Nebulizers
CPAP equipment
Braces (the kind for your limbs, not your teeth!)
Glucometers
Blood pressure monitors
Mobility devices (walkers, wheelchairs)
Infusion pumps

This small act of preparation easily eliminates a significant source of miscommunication between patients and providers.

How to Use Voice Memos

As for the voice memo feature, it never hurts to record an appointment or a discussion in order to go over what was said if you can't remember or want to do more research. It's a courteous (mandatory, really) practice to ask someone if it's all right to record them before you commence. Just explain your purpose is for your own understanding and health literacy. Providers know it's often a lot to take in, so the request should be welcome.

GENETIC TESTING: IS IT WORTH IT?

Home genetic testing falls somewhere above tarot cards and below pregnancy tests in terms of its usefulness and validity, and it is a source of confusion for many patients. To have access to information that can illuminate risk or potentially nip a fatal disease in the bud has obvious appeal. Many of us, myself included, are asking if it's worth it.

Of course, some tests *are* indeed warranted and provide meaningful information. These include, but are not limited to, the tests for Huntington's (when it runs in the family), the BRCA1 and BRCA2 genes (which are closely linked to hereditary breast cancers), and possibly neurotransmitter synthesis like the cyp450 test (which affects antidepressant therapy — see page 160). These are primarily done under the supervision of a medical provider. The rest of this section discusses other forms of genetic home testing.

Bioinformatics is a burgeoning field, a seventh wonder in the world of medicine — but also one with a nefarious past steeped in eugenics. Today it's the new darling of the start-up industry, with companies touting lifestyle DNA analyses that sound like headlines from the *Onion:* find out your cellular age, your preferences in wine, your future child's athletic abilities.

If you feel like home genetic testing promises more than it could possibly deliver, you're correct. If you get your hands on an at-home genetic testing kit, you'll see that the companies who make them are also self-conscious of this fact, their fine print rife with disclaimers. Nevertheless, companies like 23andMe and Helix (dubbed the Apple of bioinformatics) are carving out a multibillion-dollar industry. A branch of their products offers patients a hands-on way to assess their risk for certain diseases and adjust their habits accordingly. All they have to do is spit in a vial or draw a drop of blood from their index finger and mail it out to a lab.

But the results of these tests are predominantly inconclusive. Much of the time, in exchange for their saliva patients receive results that read "VUS": "variant of unknown/uncertain significance." Our DNA is rife with variation because our cells divide close to two trillion times a day, and every division is an opportunity for mutation. And even if your results show a mutation linked to breast cancer, or Alzheimer's, or ALS (Lou Gehrig's disease), it's only a matter of probability whether the mutation will indeed end up expressing itself as disease. It's like a tornado warning — the necessary conditions may be present, but no one can say for sure whether the tornado will hit your home, your neighbor's, or nobody's at all.

Interpretation

Another problem with home genetic tests is that there aren't many viable outlets in clinical care to handle the powerful information (of questionable validity) the tests reveal. As more and more tests slip into our line of sight, we become more convinced that we need them, not realizing that the results may confuse, falsely reassure, or instill in us unfounded panic. This panic then lands back on the medical system, as genetic-testing companies slyly assume a "not it" position when it comes to interpreting results beyond the molecular level. Troubling results come with an asterisk that directs you to go see your general practitioner to discuss further — and the company makes it someone else's problem.

When genetic tests yield a conclusive result about disease risk, they advise having the test repeated at your clinic or hospital with your primary care provider. But if you show up at an appointment with your results in hand, your provider may respond with skepticism or befuddlement. It can be difficult for clinicians to interpret findings in a meaningful way or come up with an actionable plan. It's also unlikely that insurance will cover a series of tests set in motion by a self-ordered testing kit, and tests are much more expensive inside the medical system, where protocol differs. Ultimately, there's not yet recourse or functional avenues for home genetic testing in the medical system. And without a way to act on or contextualize this information, I doubt it's worthwhile.

Counseling

If you do go ahead with testing, what do you do with genetic information once you have it? Aside from trying to make sense of your genome and any risks you may have uncovered, you'll need another source of help that outsourced testing universally lacks — counseling. Making sense of test results and navigating the decisions that follow can be agonizing if a grave disease is on the table. Clinics and hospitals have departments devoted to coaching patients and providers through this process, from deciding whether to have testing in the first place, to assessing results, to deciding what precautions are necessary.

And here is where I reiterate the importance of your PCP. Why not begin this process with a provider you trust at the helm, and an advisory board of genetic specialists? Rather than opening a Pandora's box of information, any possible strand of which could perplex you rather than inform or protect you, tailor a plan based on your individual risk profile with the help of a medical professional you know well.

I say skip the mail-order tests and use the money on a year of massages.

SHOULD I GOOGLE MY SYMPTOMS?

If you head for the Internet to substantiate your dread or grant peace of mind whenever you have a strange rash or something in the toilet looks unrecognizable, you're like most modern patients.

About 1 percent of all Google searches are related to medical symptoms. Google's platform for generating results for these queries isn't perfect, but they've started to refine it, working with Harvard Medical School and the Mayo Clinic to improve search results. For now, though, the Internet is best used when you need simple medical information *urgently.* Things like, *What temperature indicates that a newborn needs to go to the ER?* Or, *What are the signs and symptoms of a stroke?*

To use the Internet to your advantage for more complex medical questions, pay attention to the quality of sources you're clicking on. I recommend circumventing the whole Google affair here, because with it you're likely to be ambushed with ads and waylaid by information of dubious quality.

Instead, start with the US National Library of Medicine (http://nlm.nih.gov). The home page has several helpful branches for patients, but for your purposes MedlinePlus is the first one to click on. MedlinePlus takes research from the National Library of Medicine and distills it into information accessible on a broad range of educational levels. PubMed, a database of medical information updated in real time around the world, is the next step up. Nearly all research published in peer-reviewed health journals can be found via this database, and the bulk is accessible to the public free of charge. These articles can be daunting, so go for the abstract (a condensed paragraph that summarizes the article) or skip straight to the conclusion to find what you need.

If you do stick with Google because it's what you know and prefer, make sure the sites you end up on have a date. If the site is not from the current year, the information is likely outdated. Also check whether the author is identifiable and whether the site is sponsored by ads — particularly for medications or drug companies.

Last, monitor your state of mind when you search your symptoms. Don't do it when you're panicked or desperate, or have low blood sugar. Your frame of mind will shape the information you find and how you proceed with it. What's your endgame? Try to decide beforehand whether you want to entrust the matter to yourself and the World Wide Web, or whether you plan to see a provider anyway. If you move forward with your search, watch out for confirmation bias. If you sit down to your computer thinking, "I have skin cancer," do not type in "DO I HAVE SKIN CANCER?" because you're priming the Internet to tell you, yes, you do indeed! Instead, enter in specifics about the mole or rash, use PubMed, or go to the Skin Cancer Foundation site and read about manifestations of and risk factors for skin cancer from a more objective, holistic vantage point.

STAY ON NODDING TERMS WITH REALITY

We live in a frenetic world where it's easy to slip into a trance of exceptionalism and think, *It won't happen to me.*

The reverse side, of course, is understanding that the world is unpredictable and life is absurd, that our bodies function independently from our wishes and often assert their alliance to randomness alone. This mind-set is more realistic, but it, too, can reinforce a belief that there's no use in planning for health unknowns — considering them as inevitable as they are unpredictable. It invites us to take a back seat and entrust the decisions to others if and when there's a serious medical occasion.

But it takes only a tiny bit of planning to ensure that if an overwhelming medical situation transpires, you don't just move along a conveyor belt at the whim of strangers'

146

decision-making. The following sections will show you how to face tasks that will trigger dread before they impart peace. But in planning for the unexpected, you can enjoy the calm that comes with knowing that should a medical emergency happen, you and those around you are prepared with a blueprint.

CHOOSE AN ER

When it comes to trauma, not all hospitals and emergency rooms are created equal. Trauma centers are designated by local municipalities and verified by the American College of Surgeons based on indicators like resources, policies, readiness, and patient-care outcomes.

A Level I trauma center is a comprehensive care facility capable of treating every aspect of traumatic injury in an emergency. These have the best equipment, treatment modalities, and expertise, and in a crisis they're the ERs you want to end up in. On the other end of the spectrum are Level V trauma centers, which are capable of providing initial evaluation, making diagnoses, and prepping patients to be transferred to higher levels of care. They are not where you want to show up after a major accident.

This ranking system allows emergency responders to divert patients according to severity and type of trauma, but it's also useful to keep track yourself. Hospitals, especially private ones, market their certifications, but you can also go to the American Trauma Society website (http://www.amtrauma.org) and search for trauma centers by proximity to your home or work. Similarly, the Joint Commission designates stroke centers and comprehensive cardiac centers based on their ability to swiftly and expertly manage urgent manifestations of these conditions. These centers are where to go first in the event of a stroke or heart attack.

To cover your bases, locate the places you would go in your town or city for different emergencies, and keep a list of them accessible somewhere in the kitchen.

ADVANCE DIRECTIVES

In nursing school we had one afternoon-long lecture on advance directives, a topic that sounded so dry most skipped class that day. My friend Lilly and I sat in the back row for what turned out to be a stirring talk on the scenarios we choose not to think about, and the realities that befall both patients and medical professionals when people neglect to plan for them. By the end of the class, we'd agreed to be each other's medical decision makers, or surrogates, in the event of a medical crisis. I think I made her swear, among other things, to get my dog, and I promised her I'd never let them send the hospice harpist into her room. Lilly is loyal, sharp, and reliably capable in a crisis. She has big brown eyes and can look anything in the face without flinching — I knew there was no one I'd rather advocate for me if I couldn't do it myself.

When we fail to plan for misfortune, namely medical misfortune, we place gravely personal decisions in the hands of a stranger or, worse, a partner, sibling, or friend already in considerable distress.

There are three separate documents you need to know about to ensure these decisions aren't reactive but are rather a reflection of your preferences and wishes: the living will, the healthcare power of attorney, and the POLST.

Living Will

The living will is a legal document that lays out what interventions you would want if you were unable to make your own medical decisions, and where you would draw the proverbial line. It asks, for example, whether you would want the following:

Artificial breathing via machine
Artificial nutrition via feeding tube
Treatment that might hasten decline but
keep you comfortable

The document can be drawn up with the guidance of a lawyer (the cost is typically $1,000–$2,000), but you can find free templates online and in most local clinics and hospitals. (These must be notarized to be legally binding. Notaries typically charge $5–$10.) If you already have a relationship with a lawyer or you have complex health issues, work with a professional to draft this will. If you don't fall into these categories, it's perfectly sufficient to go the more economical route. The types of living wills that hold up in court vary from state to state, so if you split the year between New York and Florida, draft two.

Keep in mind as you make your decisions that refusing aggressive treatment, such as artificial life support, does *not* translate to refusing care to keep you comfortable, such as pain medication.

Healthcare Power of Attorney
In this document, you'll appoint someone who will make complex medical decisions for you in an unanticipated emergency —

for instance, to move forward with a high-risk procedure or persist with life-sustaining treatment for a given period of time. This individual should be someone you trust, and someone with moral courage. (For some, it's easier to designate a non–family member.) While this document stands on its own and cannot be looped into a living will, it's best to create and adapt them in tandem.

POLST

The POLST (the name varies from state to state, but generally means "physician orders for life-sustaining treatment") is a free medical document that should be signed with a provider. This is for adults who face a terminal diagnosis, or who are elderly and frail. In its most basic form, it is the standard of care when, for instance, a heart stops, for clinicians to do everything possible to save a life. This sounds good on paper, but the reality can be harsh: Picture, for instance, a frail elderly woman with terminal cancer who goes into cardiac arrest and receives CPR by the responders. Unlike in the movies, real CPR can mean broken ribs, a cracked sternum, collapsed lungs, and an electric shock to the heart. She might suffer significantly from these complications, even if they do keep her heart beating. The POLST form allows her to decide on the level of intervention she wants and the risks she'll accept.

The most important things to remember about the above forms are:

They work together and do not replace each other.

They are not set in stone and can be altered at any time.

You should share them with family and close friends.

You should have copies of each on file with your primary care doctor.

Rebecca Solnit writes, "Afraid of the darkness of the unknown, the spaces in which we see only dimly, we often choose the darkness of closed eyes." It's instinctive to close our eyes and avert our attention when it comes to imagining the worst. In spite of this, channel your guts. Gather your friends, get out the good whiskey, and make a party of it. Go around the Thanksgiving table and ask family members if they've done it. Be a model for your neighbors and coworkers. You might find that rather than being an unhappy task, it opens doors to enriching conversations with the people who make up your life.

FIVE:
DRUGS 101

DRUG NOMENCLATURE

Here is a short-and-sweet, easy-to-remember concept that will give you an advantage when navigating your health: Every drug has *two* names — the trade or brand name and the generic name (a mouthful based on the drug's molecular structure). If you've ever heard your provider refer to a medication you're taking with an unfamiliar name, this is why. Because medical jargon isn't already confounding enough, we've thrown in one more element of confusion. Here are a few examples:

Trade/brand name — Generic name:
Lexapro — escitalopram
Nexium — esomeprazole
Plavix — clopidogrel bisulfate

Knowing both names of the medications

you're prescribed and the over-the-counter medications you take regularly will not only ease participation in conversations with your providers, but it will also amplify your ability to fend off medical error, which we'll get to later.

Knowing both names can also help you save money at the drugstore. When you're trying to choose between three packages of a similar medication, you can look at the ingredient list and know exactly what you're dealing with! Every drug in branded packaging also has the generic name listed, while bottles dispensed by a pharmacist tend to only use the generic name. A quick Google search of "generic name for [x]" will get you what you need. A comprehensive list of both names of every drug can be found at http://www.rxlist.com.

HAVE A HEADACHE?

Ibuprofen, Motrin, Tylenol, Advil. We keep them stocked in our medicine cabinets and store bottles in our handbags. (One time I even woke up next to someone who kept them in a glass jar, like M&M's, on their nightstand for hangovers.) These anti-inflammatory drugs are the workhorse in our modern apothecary, but like any medication, they can have severe side effects.

Here are seemingly random but important things to remember when taking these over-the-counter drugs.

Aspirin (acetylsalicylic acid) is its own animal, since its chemical makeup is distinct from those of other painkillers we take regularly. It's an acid and a blood thinner, so many people take a "baby dose" daily when they have a high risk for heart disease.

- When aspirin travels through the stomach, it thins the special layer of mucus that protects the stomach from acid, increasing the risk for bleeding.
- Aspirin can also be toxic to the ears, causing tinnitus, or ringing — a sign that you have taken too much.
- It is contraindicated (should never be used) for a child or adolescent with a respiratory illness (cold or flu) or chicken pox, as it can cause a dangerous condition called Reye's syndrome.
- Because aspirin is a blood thinner, mixing it with alcohol or anticoagulants (such as Plavix or warfarin) will increase the risk of bleeding.
- If an aspirin bottle smells like yeast or

vinegar, it has lost its potency. Throw it out!

Nonselective NSAIDS (e.g., ibuprofen/ Advil and Motrin, naproxen/Aleve) are anti-inflammatory, pain relieving, and fever reducing. (NSAID stands for "nonsteroidal anti-inflammatory drug.")

- They take one to two hours to relieve pain and two to four hours to bring down a fever. Keep this timeline in mind so you don't take another dose while waiting for the first to peak. If you use them to bring down inflammation from a chronic disease like arthritis, it will take one to two weeks for results to manifest.
- This particular group of drugs is not ideal for older adults, as they pose a risk of fatal ulcers in this population. They are also not a good option for people struggling with diabetes, heart failure, cirrhosis, hemophilia, or ulcers, or who are taking lithium.
- When these NSAIDS are used in excess over the course of a life, they increase the risk of hypertension, heart attack, and stroke, so don't pop them with abandon!

156

Acetaminophen (Tylenol) does not have an anti-inflammatory effect because it works on the central nervous system rather than the peripheral nervous system.

- Because it works centrally, Tylenol is a good alternative for elderly or pregnant patients. It's also a good option if you're prone to ulcers.
- At high doses it can be damaging to the liver, which is why a Tylenol overdose can be fatal or necessitate a liver transplant if it's not reversed with an antidote within eight hours.

POLYPHARMACY

Doctors pour medicines about which they know little, for diseases about which they know less, into human beings about whom they know nothing.

— VOLTAIRE

Medications are a gift of modern medicine, but it's easy to have too much of a good thing. As soon as there are lots of different meds on board (called "polypharmacy"), they're bound to start causing problems of their own, either by taxing your body's system or by interacting with one another.

For example, chronic conditions tend to come with a cabinet full of different medications: One for the pain. Another for the side effect the first medication causes. Another for a separate symptom that came about from the first two clashing. In balancing the many aspects of a chronic illness, providers run the risk of prescribing too many medications. This can include ones that aren't necessary or that cancel each other out when taken together. It's especially likely to happen with adults who struggle with more than one chronic illness and must navigate interventions for both.

Problems related to polypharmacy can include:

Taking medications for a symptom when in fact they're not helping it

Treating one illness with multiple equivalent medications

Using medications that interact with each other

Using an inappropriate dose

Treating adverse drug reactions with other medications

Most healthcare providers have yet to master the art of successfully deprescribing. Studies have shown that most operate on the general principle that the benefits of a drug outweigh the risks; they are also overwhelmingly unaware that they're over-prescribing. Providers are generally inclined to keep you on a medication they believe will help your underlying condition, and then treat its side effects accordingly. Even for those who do want to deprescribe, there's a dearth of research to help them figure out how to do it best. The majority of studies are about what happens when patients *take* a drug, not what happens when they stop taking it.

Polypharmacy and its negative effects have to be treated on a case-by-case basis. There are no tests you can run to see what's interacting, and when you're taking several medications with overlapping side effects it's difficult to sleuth out which med is causing what symptom. It's an area of medicine that requires skill and excellent communication between providers and patients.

A few examples of symptoms that can arise from polypharmacy:

Confusion
Weakness
Tremors
Hair loss
Incontinence

Sensory deficits
Fainting

The worst of the worst!

It's not unusual to leave an appointment with a new prescription, or leave a hospital stay with a boatload of new medications. These are opportune times to reassess your medication list in full with the prescriber. At each routine exam, visit with a specialist, or hospital discharge, be sure to ask this question: *Can we cut anything?*

When you are taking several medications for one condition or syndrome, any new symptom might actually be a side effect. If you have a chronic illness and take multiple medications, it's important to tune in to changes in your body in the first two weeks after starting any new medication. In your notebook or using a symptom tracker app, like Symple, take a moment each day to note any changes you're experiencing in appetite, sleep, mood, or bowel movement, including things as subtle as malaise or general lethargy.

ANTIDEPRESSANTS

Antidepressants are prescribed more liberally today than ever before. Prozac hit the American scene in the late eighties, and today one in ten adults takes an antidepressant, with over fifty different types to choose from. And you no longer need to lie on a leather chaise longue and divulge your feelings to get one — primary care providers write scripts for them.

Though I advocate for having a primary mental healthcare provider and supplementing with therapy (see page 95), it's fine to work with a primary care provider to find the right medication if it's convenient and feels right to you. That said, it's important to consider that most general practitioners (like your family doctor) don't have extensive training in antidepressant therapy, which is a nascent field and more of an art than an exact science.

No matter who you work with, the first medication you try will simply be an educated guess on the part of the provider. Brain chemistry varies infinitely. Neurotransmission is a complicated dance, and it requires finesse and patience, trial and error, to find the right treatment.

Here are some things to guide you in finding the medication(s) you'll respond to best:

Approach with patience. I remind patients every day that it can take trials with two, three, or four medications before finding the right one. Pay attention to your body and mood carefully in the first few weeks, and schedule a follow-up call or appointment to assess things with your provider. Request this even if it's not automatically offered or scheduled.

To avoid enduring so many trials, consider asking your provider about a cytochrome p450 test. This is a simple cheek swab that analyzes your genetic ability to metabolize medications. It may guide the provider in choosing the medication and the dose, and help them avoid medications to which you could have an adverse or blunted reaction.*

If you have tried several antidepressants without noticeable improvement of symptoms, ask your provider about a methylation test. This relatively new, noninvasive genetic test will determine how much folate you metabolize and absorb. Folic acid (a derivative of folate)

* Disclaimer: The research on the effectiveness of these tests is new and somewhat conflicting, but broach the topic with your provider and make the decision for yourself.

is necessary to synthesize neurotransmitters like serotonin and dopamine that play key roles in balancing our mood and behavior. Antidepressants can't work well for you if you don't metabolize folate — it would be like trying to make meringue without egg whites! The solution is as simple as taking a supplement.

■ ■ ■ ■

Part II
When It's Routine

■ ■ ■ ■

Routine appointments with your primary care provider are an ideal space to practice exercising your agency. The issues bringing you in are typically low stakes — physicals, vaccines, health screenings for employers or universities. They're also valuable because they provide face time, giving you a chance to build a relationship with your primary care provider and hit a stride in how you communicate with them.

The following sections will guide you through the natural trajectory of a routine appointment, from intake to follow-up. They will cover the art of scheduling appointments, intake and what we tend to gloss over during intake, and how to talk to your provider.

Six:
Making Your Way into the System

Tricks of Scheduling Appointments

There's an art to scheduling appointments: part grace, part insight.

I spent summers as a medical receptionist before I went to nursing school, and I've found that a few small considerations will go a long way to scheduling appointments:

For routine appointments, opt for spring and summer months. Other patients are away on vacation, and it's generally easier to get in when you'd like to.

Unless you have a pressing issue, you might avoid scheduling anything routine during the winter months — cold and flu season. Going to the clinic then means exposing yourself to an army of germs better left in their waiting-room cesspool and not on your person.

167

If you're expecting to discuss specific lab results at your appointment, call the office ahead of time and make sure the results are in. If they aren't, reschedule.

If there's the option, try for appointments no later than 1 p.m. to avoid residual, end-of-day wait times.

If you have a very strict schedule, call the office the day of your appointment to see if things are on schedule. If they're behind, ask when to show up.

There will, of course, be moments for which you can't plan, when you'll need an appointment with a provider you know ASAP. Like if you have a shooting pain in your back for which your PCP has given you a cortisone shot in the past, and it suddenly reemerges when you're at the office. Regrettably, you can't holler, *Someone fetch the doctor, quick!* and wait for them to arrive with their black bag. But a same-day appointment isn't out of the question — even in this day and age of exceedingly booked clinics and strapped providers. It takes a little strategy and a bit of finessing, but it can be done:

Call between the hours of 10:30 and 11 a.m. It's after the morning bustle, and a golden hour for cancellations.

When you call, do not leave a message. Instead, try a few times until you get a human being on the phone.

If your issue can be handled over the phone (for example, you need advice about the severity of something, a prescription called in, or a referral), ask the person on the other end of the phone if the provider would be amenable to a phone call, or if you can email or text them. (This flexibility is something to consider when choosing your PCP. See page 77 on "What to Look For.") If you're trying to get general advice, talk to a nurse first. See if they can advise.

Wednesdays, on the whole, tend to be the slowest days with the most openings.

Mondays and Fridays should be a last resort. Mondays are the busiest; on Fridays, most staff try to scoot out early, and they want to lighten their schedule rather than add to it.

Dress Up for Better Care

Without fail, my mother always reminded us to wear our finest undies when we went to the pediatrician. Sometimes she even bought us new ones. I never understood this practice and hadn't thought about it in years, until I came across a *Forbes* article that proposed that patients who dress up receive better healthcare and are more likely to have their concerns acknowledged. Dressing well is a power move in other professional and life arenas, so it makes sense.

From the moment you step into a medical setting, doctors and nurses are appraising you — subtly, often unconsciously, assessing your appearance, hygiene, cognitive state, body language, and the way you move about the world. We are trained to notice. If you dress up (and by this I mean something thoughtful, not black tie!), even just a little bit, it gives the impression you're taking things seriously. When you show up for an appointment looking spiffy, it suggests your day involves ritual. It says — even if in the most understated way — you value yourself, the exchange, and your health.

If these reasons don't move you to go find a silk ascot or monkstrap shoes, consider doing it for yourself. Research shows that dressing up helps you feel confident and competent, and these are definitely states to channel at appointments. Unless you feel like death warmed over, give this rule a try and see how it goes. Wear something your grandmother would say you look smart in. You might be surprised by the difference.

WHILE YOU WAIT

Waiting rooms invite you to check out while the time passes, and they have ample sources of distraction: books, games, last June's issue of *Cosmopolitan.*

About a year ago I started challenging myself not to dive into my phone, or pick up whatever book is in my bag, when I take up residence in a waiting room. Without an intentional pause, the inertia of the day follows me right into the room and I'm more detached and distracted when the appointment finally begins.

If waiting for an appointment to start puts you in the throes of panic — or even if you're the type of person who can shift from the outside world to inside the exam room with agility — take this moment of quiet to prepare. If you're nervous, find a place in your body that feels relaxed or solid and place your attention on it. Reflect on what you want to cover when you head back there. The point is to subtly prepare yourself

171

to shift gears, to make sure your mind and body can get in sync and line up for the appointment, where they are both needed in equal measure.

Allergies

Every time you check in at a clinic, urgent care facility, or hospital room, someone in scrubs will ask you — yet again — if you have any allergies. Even if you just wrote it down on the form they're holding.

They do this because missing or incorrectly interpreting a patient's allergies is a major source of error in the medical world. Results of such errors can range from minor (hives) to fatal (anaphylaxis). And these aren't just rookie mistakes made by residents and nursing students: seasoned practitioners succumb to them, in the operating room and while prescribing.

Without placing all the blame on technology, allergy-related error is a prime example of what happens when electronic medical records and their endless checkboxes prime clinicians to turn on autopilot. It's understandable when they ask the question one hundred times a day. You'll need to accentuate your humanness and jolt them out of it!

Here are a few quick things to remember

172

the next time you encounter this broken record of a question:

If you have serious allergies, state them and then ask, "Can I see my chart to make sure they're entered correctly?" Even if you can infer from the original question that they were, it sets a precedent. It makes everyone stand up a little straighter, look at you instead of the screen, and pay better attention, because of the importance you're assigning to the matter.

When you're regurgitating your list of allergies, you will be asked, "And what happens when you're exposed to it?" Be clear in your answer. If you get a rash every time you eat shrimp, it's not necessary to expound upon, but if, for instance, you've had a reaction to codeine that necessitated medical intervention, describe what happened in detail.

Antibiotics are a common allergen. If you're allergic to penicillin, you could be allergic to a handful of other antibiotics in the penicillin family. If you're ever prescribed something ending in "-cillin" (see "Antibiotics" for reference), notify

173

the prescriber about your allergy and confirm that the drug is safe for you.

If you're ever prescribed something you're allergic to, do not take it. Do not assume everyone knows what they're doing; assume your allergy was overlooked.

This may only apply to a fraction of readers, but if you've ever had Stevens-Johnson syndrome in reaction to a medication, mention it up front and emphatically during every medical encounter. Never retake a drug that caused this effect, even if you're told it's safe.

Vitamins and Supplements

Intake forms tend to drag on. They nag you to answer personal questions, and they're repetitive. It's easy to breeze through them, but be sure to pay attention to the questions about current medications — including vitamins, supplements, and over-the-counter drugs.

While they may appear mild compared to prescriptions, vitamins and supplements are indeed potent! Saint-John's-wort, sometimes used for depression, can counteract the effects of certain allergy medications. Garlic supplements thin the blood and increase the risk of postsurgical bleeding. Echinacea, which has potent effects on the immune system, should be avoided while pregnant or breastfeeding. Valerian, kava, and chamomile, while helpful for a good night's sleep, intensify certain side effects of opioids. Dandelion and juniper have strong antioxidant properties, but they also act as diuretics and can affect the kidneys. Licorice root (or even copious amounts of black licorice candy) mimics a hormone called aldosterone, which regulates blood pressure.

Your providers need to know about everything on board. So whether you've meddled in the black magic of natural remedies or you live far from the equator and take vitamin D, list every last vitamin and supplement on the good old intake form.

MAKING THE MOST OF YOUR TIME AT APPOINTMENTS

If you have a nagging feeling that you're being rushed during every medical encounter, it's not in your head. The average length of an appointment is seven to nine minutes. You can circumvent this issue by choosing a practice or provider that's more accessible (see "What to Look For," page 77), but one-on-one time is almost always in short supply. Appointments leave most patients reeling, with a sinking sense they've only touched the tip of the iceberg in the short conversation.

This means that winging it during your appointment won't be the best use of your time. Providers will guide you along and ask the questions they need to ask, but if you don't prepare ahead it might take you five appointments to cover everything you want to talk about. But with just a bit of forethought and planning, you can reasonably address it all in one conversation.

Before heading in, whether it's for a routine checkup or a surfacing health issue, make a list of the things you need to get across during your allotted time with your provider. Do you need vaccinations? Do you want to talk about screenings relevant to your age group? Do you need a referral? What maintenance and health-promotion issues do you want you bring up?

THE INTAKE CONVERSATION

Jostle Robots

Routine encounters can take place in one of three ways. Some medical professionals will enter like a beam of light and make you feel like the only person in the room. Some will rock back and forth between you and the screen. And the last bunch might look at you only when they enter and exit the room, with a medical scribe on a laptop trailing them.

Over the last decade, electronic medical record (EMR) systems have become ubiquitous. And when it comes to EMRs, the first goal is not communication, it's checking off boxes. This is not always a bad thing. It ensures a more rigid, streamlined system that often prevents error. Where a provider might once have waltzed through a nurses' station and said, "LOL [little old lady] in room six needs ten milligrams of propranolol, stat," or passed the request on via a note written in frantic chicken scratch that caused the nurse to read "1.0 milligrams" instead of "10," they now enter it in a system, ensuring that everyone is on the same page.

For practitioners, EMRs streamline the process of collecting information. But using them can be a menial and rote activity, and they may nod off or miss something. Studies have demonstrated that pen-to-paper writing and computer typing involve vastly different cognitive processes, and the neural underpinnings of face-to-face communication fall into another category altogether. The take-home message: When the system was overhauled to use solely electronic records, important modes of communication were lost.

This hit me one day at a patient intake. I asked the next question on my screen, which was about family history:

Are there significant health conditions in your immediate family?

My brother has asthma, and my dad had a stent placed in 2008.

Okay, and Mom?

She died from lung cancer.

Age of death?

Still staring at the screen, I would have kept going had she not paused for a good thirty seconds, causing me to look up. She explained that her mom had died the month prior at the age of fifty-five. The patient was at a physical she'd waited too long to cancel. Through more discussion, it came out that she was getting two to three hours of sleep per night and felt isolated in a debilitating depression — which I don't think she would have shared if I'd kept thoughtlessly scrolling through questions.

Another time, I went with a friend to an appointment and watched her discomfort as the nurse asked her the same routine family-history questions. Adopted from Korea as a baby, my friend knew nothing about her biological family's medical history, but she tolerated the inquisition without interrupting, out of politeness. And the nurse just kept going, clicking for every relative.

Why was her nurse acting like a robot? Why had I? The glaring downside to technology is that it puts us on autopilot. Intakes become a host of boxes to tick, and even when the questions are open-ended, we miss crucial information from body language and eye contact because we are furiously typing away, trying to capture everything the patient says.

Technology has turned much of the communication in exam rooms two- rather than three-dimensional, rendering it problematic and certainly less therapeutic. There's a reason it's uncouth to break up with someone over text, a reason you write your grandfather a card rather than send an email.

If I'd kept on with the form, my patient might not have disclosed her depression or insomnia. If the provider took the intake notes from my friend's nurse at face value, they could have assumed that she was just a fortunate patient who didn't carry much genetic risk.

Checkboxes don't capture nuance. Healthcare providers are coming up with creative solutions to address this, but in the meantime it's important for patients to understand their limitations. You might have to lean into your social graces during this part of your appointment. If an open-ended question comes up or a usually routine question warrants more than a one-sentence answer, pause and preface it with something like:

This is complicated, so I want to be sure I explain it well . . .

This is something that's changed for me recently . . .

This one is always hard for me to answer because . . .

This is a jostle, a little bolt of electricity that primes the clinician to look at you and stop typing. It's a gentle reminder to listen to you.

White Lies

Have you ever bent the truth when talking to a provider? Conservatively selected "two to four" drinks per week instead of "four to eight" on the intake form? (*Red wine is full of beneficial resveratrol, so those are probably a net neutral! And "four to eight" is probably just used to identify alcoholics, anyway!*) Inversely, have you been a bit liberal in discussing your exercise habits? *I'd say about five to six times a week. Yes, indeed, getting my heart rate above one hundred every time. I'm Jane Fonda.*

Have you been evasive about your sex life, or the frequency with which you use protection? Have you made something up about the onset of your symptoms because the nurse asked, and even though you're a rather poor historian you felt a frantic need to provide useful information?

Did you fabricate a symptom you may not actually have had, but only read about on WebMD, to help the provider make a diagnosis?

Did you coolly shake your head when the pediatrician asked if you let your newborn baby sleep in the bed with you?

If any of this sounds familiar, it's because almost all of us have done it. Most patients have omitted, selectively told, or bent the truth — whether consciously or unconsciously — at some point during a clinical encounter. (Providers do it too, by the way, primarily when they have to share bad news or admit an error.) It doesn't make us bad patients, just human patients, who possess a compulsion to please authority figures — and who like to maintain a certain blindness to our own weaknesses when it comes to a healthy lifestyle.

Is there a hierarchy of deceit when it comes to little white lies to the white coat? Well, yes. Sleep is too important. If you're not getting enough and you aren't inclined to discuss that, it's the insomnia talking. Bring it up. Aside from that, I'm not going to tell you that it's never okay to keep something private and uncomfortable off the examination table.

When the tendency to paint a rosier picture comes up, though, you should stop and ask yourself where it's coming from. Tell us you're unblighted and you love kale and sure, we'll write it down in your chart. But to whose benefit is it really if it's not true?

If you drink a glass of wine every night and the occasional dirty martini on weekends, and report it honestly, your provider isn't likely to hand you rehab pamphlets. But if instead you significantly underestimate how much you drink per week, and you're a woman, your provider might miscategorize your risk for breast cancer and skip a conversation that could matter to you greatly.

If you don't work out enough, that's okay. This habit is not static. It depends on age, expendable time, and access to gyms, parks, or trails, and these fluctuate based on life circumstances. Altering your responses here might avoid a conversation, *the* conversation, that could get you exercising again or more frequently. Give your provider a chance to support or motivate you — you might be happy you did.

Next, if you cannot comply with a treatment regimen — whether it's taking a medication at specific hours of the day, sleeping with a CPAP throughout the night, or using your inhaler as prescribed — speak up. It's confounding when you continue to report symptoms but your provider is under the impression you're doing X, Y, and Z. If you know you won't follow through with a prescription, ask your provider to discuss alternatives with you. There's no need to suffer in silence while not getting benefit from a treatment.

Sometimes we evade conversations because of someone in the room other than the medical professionals. While I think you should generally avoid going to important appointments alone if you can help it, there are also cases in which someone might come with you even if you don't want them to.

When you need privacy, tell the staff when checking in that you'd like to see the provider alone first, and then your person can be called back. This is the standard procedure, for instance, at every Planned Parenthood.

In more grave circumstances, patients (usually women) might be accompanied to appointments by an abusive partner, as it's a way for the abuser to extend control. If you are in a situation of any kind and feel unsafe speaking about it during a clinical encounter because of a partner's presence, one option is to call the clinic ahead and state specifically that you're calling in confidence because your partner plans to accompany you and you need to be seen alone at the beginning of the appointment. Ask that they flag this on your chart so the team has a reminder on the day of the appointment. This can be a safe and supportive environment to discuss your situation if you do not feel comfortable doing so elsewhere.

SEVEN:
HOW TO TALK TO PROVIDERS

LOUIS WASHKANSKY AND
THE WESTERN

On December 3, 1967, Louis Washkansky, a Lithuanian-born Jew turned South African immigrant, received the world's first human-to-human heart transplant. In an operation lasting roughly six hours, Cape Town doctor Christiaan Barnard led a team of thirty surgeons (including his brother, Marius), anesthetists, and nurses in replacing Washkansky's worn, clogged heart with a twenty-five-year-old equivalent in mint condition. It had belonged to Denise Darvall. She was a young bank clerk, with a raven-black bun and deep-set eyes (I pored over the few existing photos of her in library archives one afternoon). Hit by a car while crossing the street that December day, she was pronounced brain-dead on the scene and donated an organ that would cement itself in medical history.

185

At the urging of Washkansky's longtime family physician, Christiaan Barnard set aside time before the surgery to meet with Washkansky and his wife, Anne, to discuss expectations and concerns regarding the novel procedure. Barnard recounts how he found the patient sitting up in bed reading a Western:

"Mr. Washkansky, I have come to introduce myself. We intend doing a heart transplant on you — and for this you will be admitted to my ward."

"That's fine with me. I'm ready for it," Washkansky replied.

"If you like, I can tell you what we know and don't know about this," I went on.

Washkansky nodded and waited for me to go on. He was obviously very sick, but you could see he had once been quite strong and good-looking. There were also the features of a generous man — a large mouth with the face folds of one who smiles often. He had big ears and big hands, and his eyes, gray-green — peering at me over spectacles — were waiting. So, I spoke to him.

"We know you have a heart disease for which we can do nothing more. You have had all possible treatment and you are getting no better. We can put a normal heart in you, after taking out your heart that's no longer any good, and there's a chance you can get back to normal life."

"So they told me," Washkansky replied. "I'm ready to go ahead."

His eyes remained on me with no indication he wanted to know any more. . . . As I turned to go, he began reading again. How, I wondered, could he return to pulp fiction after being suddenly cast into the greatest drama of his life? What is it about human nature that caused such a reaction? No man in the history of the world had ever met the surgeon who was going to cut out his heart and replace it with a new human one — at least, not until this moment, which was now being lost somewhere in a Western novel.

I had offered him . . . life. Yet he had not asked the odds, nor a single detail.

The surgery was a success. The heart with a young woman's past was perfusing the old man's organs as the surgeons closed up. Washkansky lived for another eighteen days, just enough time for him to sit up and speak with the press before his immune system, perplexed and overburdened, gave out. The fate was a surprise to no one: The medical team knew full well the inherent risk involved, and the reality that they themselves were entering a Wild West; the transplant was a shot in the dark, the odds in no one's favor. A surprise to no one, that is, except Washkansky, cold in the morgue, and his wife, who'd initially felt they'd been the recipients of miraculous fortune. A new beginning was, in the end, merely an encore.

Now, I'll take you back to the present. In his book *The Silent World of Doctor and Patient,* Jay Katz recounts this story of the first heart transplant as part of a discussion on informed-consent practices — particularly those of which he took a dim view, like Barnard's.

Katz's book came to me by way of a woman central to this book, Helen Haskell, in February 2018. We spent Valentine's Day on the phone, talking about this world of omissions and miscommunications between patients and medical providers. It was a world she found herself in when her teenage son died from medical error at a South Carolina hospital in 2000 (the full story lives in chapter 20). In some ways, things haven't changed, we concluded. It's still difficult to communicate with providers. We've all got a bit of Washkansky in us when it comes to unknowns in the world of medicine.

Washkansky, awaiting the first-ever heart transplant, was about to enter a heroic, unpredictable Wild West of his own, and yet he approached his predicament like the storybook in his hands. Today, patients watch medical encounters unfold around us in precisely the same way. When we cross the threshold into the healthcare world, it's easy for us to assume that medical providers are omniscient, omnipotent, and totally in control of our well-being. In turn, it's not uncommon for us to relinquish our voice and behave like characters (rather than real, flesh-and-blood, feeling people) in a narrative over which we have no control. Instead of confronting the chaotic and uncertain landscape into which we are thrown when we get sick, we often prefer, like Washkansky, to escape to fictional landscapes in which we are voyeurs rather than active participants, where the characters' fates are predetermined and the author is in control of the plot.

As modern patients we tend to watch medical encounters unfold in precisely the same way. We hand over the reins. We tamp down our voice. We count on the narrative arc. And yet when we take a back seat rather than an active role in deciding our fate within the healthcare system, it may end up determined by outside forces that are essentially ambivalent.

The crucial aspect of rewriting this story is to learn how to talk to providers. It is to learn how to ask questions so that you feel informed and confident in your medical decision-making. Whether going under for an experimental transplant or getting a Pap smear, this task is essential.

The following sections will give you a framework for how to talk to providers and will hopefully make the affair more pleasant and less intimidating. But first — now that I've forbid you to escape to fictional landscapes — we'll have to do it once more.

THE GOLDEN TENTACLE

There's a scene in F. Scott Fitzgerald's *This Side of Paradise* that stays with me. The narrator, in the throes of young love, expresses a wish to bend tiny golden tentacles from his imagination to his love interest's. I have always loved the image because it reflects those rare, sweet, satisfying moments in a conversation when you realize that you and the other person are on the same wavelength. Sometimes it feels like having a conversation with yourself. Sometimes you finish each other's sentences or jump from topic to topic in a way that makes no sense to the outside observer, but makes complete sense to the two of you. It's a transcendence born of being heard and understood. That golden tentacle is what you're aiming for at your appointments.

Hopefully you've found a PCP with whom you have a good rapport, but you can still take extra steps to ensure you communicate well. The topics we're about to discuss are geared toward any routine care appointments, but the ideas also lend themselves to communicating when something is wrong, or you have a chief complaint. They can be applied to topics in chapter 9, "Navigating Touchy Territory," as well.

THE UNIQUE ROLE OF QUESTIONS

Medical appointments can feel like interviews. Providers are trained to use algorithms and deductive reasoning to get an accurate picture of what's going on. Patients, in turn, endure the Q and A. This stiff back-and-forth is the main model we have for medical encounters. Like your average interview, it goes something like:

Exchange of pleasantries

Question and answer session
Exchange of pleasantries

But the visit should be more than comments about the weather, a brief synopsis of your health, and a *Take care, now!* at the end. An encounter with any medical professional should have more of the organic characteristics of a proper conversation.

We use questions to steer a conversation, change a topic or return to one, and help shepherd the person across from us through our thinking. Questions are a critical expression of a patient's power.

Sociolinguist Nancy Ainsworth-Vaughn dedicated the latter part of her career to examining the specific ways questions alter the course of patient care. She reviewed thousands of hours of taped conversations between patients and doctors in the late eighties and early nineties, using standardized measures of "conversational maneuvers" to identify ways patients and doctors claimed power in conversations. She followed patient cases along the care continuum, some of them for several years, and traced the ways questions in early appointments overtly changed outcomes later on.

The modern medical encounter can be a hostile environment for questions. We're less apt to ask one if we feel the listener is rushed or impatient. And even though we're told since kindergarten that there's no such thing as a dumb question, most of us are less likely to ask when we feel less knowledgeable about the subject matter than the answerer.

Questions are not just about asking for information, however; they give the listener insight into your worldview. They point toward what we value, what we find important or relevant, and what we need to know to move forward. This was the crux of Ainsworth-Vaughn's findings: Questions and answers exchanged by patient and doctor early on incited greater understanding on the part of the physician and greater trust on the part of the patient, opening channels of communication that uncovered clues essential to diagnosis and the most beneficial treatment.

Recent scientific evidence corroborates this study, demonstrating that patients asking more questions is directly correlated to improved medical outcomes. For example, hospitalized patients who ask more questions during discharge have a lower chance of returning to the hospital. Diabetic patients who ask more questions at medical consultations have lower blood pressure and better management of blood sugar when compared to controls. So, ask more questions, especially open-ended ones.

By this I don't mean that you should conjure up queries during your appointment to fill empty space or sound intelligent. But do raise your hand whenever you have a genuine question. These might include, *Why do you say X and not Y? What would it feel like if I were experiencing X? What is the plan when I walk out the door today?*

If you don't understand why the provider is asking you a particular question, ask. If the provider's line of thinking confuses you, ask them to explain it.

You can also use a question to rein a conversation back in when you realize it's gone totally off course. If you notice the person across from you spinning off in a direction that indicates they didn't hear or understand you, don't assume your concern isn't relevant. It's okay to bring them back in by saying something like:

I might have miscommunicated this, but X is the biggest issue for me, and the thing that brought me in. Can we back up?

When receiving instructions, new prescriptions, referrals, or tests, ask yourself the following:

What is the problem?

What do I need to do about it now?

Why is it important that I do this?

What comes next?

If you don't know the answer to one of these questions, ask for elaboration. If you're worried that you might not remember, write it down in a notebook. If medical staff speak over you, impale you with too much information at once, or deliver information in a way that's not accessible to you, they're not fulfilling an important part of their job. It's okay to ask for clarification. The best providers and nurses use the teach-back method, asking you to answer these questions in front of them. They do this to ensure *they* explained things adequately.

Next, think about how you like to take in new information. Do you need to see something drawn out for it to make sense? Do you prefer to listen or read? Are you likely to read up on something or do you want the bare minimum given to you straight? Many struggle with health literacy because information is transferred in a medium that doesn't fit their learning styles. Luckily (and because there is a mass global initiative to improve health literacy in care delivery right now) hospitals and clinics will now ask on your intake paperwork how you prefer to receive information, so if verbal explanation isn't your style, they can offer alternatives. If you know you're not going to read through printed sheets, they may have videos, web resources, and pamphlets on hand to aid your learning. If this question doesn't come up on intake, let the provider know during your appointment that you'd like other learning resources and materials.

STORIES: GIVING YOURSELF CONTEXT

Storytelling claims power. No more important claim to power could be imagined than that which aims to co-construct a diagnosis (entailing treatment) and at the same time define who we are and who we will be.
— NANCY AINSWORTH-VAUGHN

Don't Go in Blind: There's Not Enough Time

During medical encounters, establishing your identity by sharing stories that give you context and celebrate your personality is a power move. When implemented effectively, stories remind everyone around you you're a human with a past, present, and future. You incite more investment from your medical staff and increase the likelihood that you will receive patient-centered care — care that carefully considers and respects each symptom, condition, or illness manifestation as pieces of your life.

Your provider's window into your life can be as large or small as you make it. The more you contextualize and shed light on who you are, the less likely you'll be to get lost in the shuffle and the more likely you'll be to get attentive, generous care. Ample research shows that making yourself seem more human invokes greater empathy from care providers. The more insistent you are about being yourself, the more relatable you'll be, the more they'll attune to you.

Does this mean you should waylay your doctor or nurse with a chapter of your memoir every time they enter the room? No, don't! But you should feel free to be yourself. Share stories when they're relevant, provide information that gives you context, allude to the people, places, and things outside the office that give your life meaning.

When the provider comes in and asks, "Hi, how are you?" take it as an opportunity instead of just saying, "I'm fine."

Say, instead, something like:

I rushed here from work, so I'm a little

frazzled. I'm an elementary school teacher, and it was a busy day.

Great! I just biked here, and it's beautiful out.

My dog is at the vet, so it's been a day.

These all give you context, and who knows — your provider may be a parent. A cyclist. A dog lover, just like you.

PART III
MAKING THE MOST
OF EACH MEDICAL
ENCOUNTER

■ ■ ■ ■

Illness is the night-side of life, a more onerous citizenship. Everyone who is born holds dual citizenship, in the kingdom of the well and in the kingdom of the sick. Although we all prefer to use only the good passport, sooner or later each of us is obliged, at least for a spell, to identify ourselves as citizens of that other place.

— SUSAN SONTAG, *ILLNESS AS METAPHOR*

The merest schoolgirl, when she falls in love, has Shakespeare or Keats to speak her mind for her; but let a sufferer try to describe a pain in his head to a doctor and language at once runs dry. There is nothing ready made for him. He is forced to coin words himself, and, taking his pain in one hand, and a lump of pure sound in the other (as perhaps the people of Babel did in the beginning), so to crush them together that a brand new word in the end drops out. Probably it will be something laughable.

— VIRGINIA WOOLF, *ON BEING ILL*

EIGHT:
WHEN SOMETHING IS WRONG

The chief complaint, now often referred to by providers as the "presenting concern," is the center on which most medical encounters will focus. It's the answer to that most essential question: "What brings you in today?"

Most of us spout off a list of symptoms in no particular order, scattered across a vague timeline. This might be because it's nerve-racking to be put on the spot, or because the problem is a blur we haven't had time to work through in our minds.

It's helpful to create a narrative or story around the situation prior to going to the appointment. This will give your symptoms context and provide meaning to the timeline, and you'll naturally equip your provider with key information you may not even realize is relevant.

Take a few notes in the comfort of your own home before you get on unfamiliar turf. The evening before your appointment, so it's fresh in your mind, write down the main bullet points for what you're going to share with your provider when they give you the floor. You might even want to practice the little talk on someone you know, ideally your advocate (see "Choosing an Advocate," beginning on page 112).

It may sound like I'm setting you up for a stiff, choreographed interaction, but the appointment should be anything but! Think of this preparation as scaffolding for a conversation. It will spare you the heartache and frustration of a wasted appointment that you leave wondering what, exactly, was accomplished.

CREATING AN ELEVATOR COMPLAINT

The art of the "elevator complaint" — a short, eloquent story about what ails you — requires you to be detailed but not exhaustive, both thorough and concise. Trim down your notes about your symptoms to the most essential. Watch out for things that may invite a long digression into your history, and parse out extraneous topics that relate only insofar as they have to do with your body and you're on an exam bench. Do you need a flu shot? Want to know when you're due for your next pelvic exam? Want to change a medication to a generic version? Save these sundry points to cover at the end of the appointment. It might seem reasonable to list off every ache and pain you've experienced from the cradle to your 9 a.m. appointment while you've got your provider's attention, but don't make elephants out of flies. Listing multiple complaints creates noise, and diagnosis is about limiting the noise. It's also liable to send you on a wild-goose chase through the medical system. The elevator complaint is the place to execute focus.

Try to pare your list of complaints down to two to four symptoms that are most pressing, or are impacting the quality of your days most intensely.

For each symptom, include the following information:

Onset (when did it start?)
Frequency
What aggravates it
Typical duration
What alleviates it
Any remedies you've tried that didn't work

If you're feeling stuck, try some of the following phrases (also see page 259 for help describing pain):

_____ (*days/weeks/months*) ago I started experiencing _____.

This symptom (*is unremitting/comes and goes/lasts for weeks at a time/is unbearable for thirty minutes, then resolves/is the same severity every time/fluctuates in severity*).

This was (*followed by/accompanied by*) _____.

The symptom is (*like when you get motion sickness/sudden and shooting like a pinched nerve*), not (*like an upset stomach before you throw up/dull like a stomachache*).

The symptom (*is worse/seems to flare up*) when _____.

I've tried (*over-the-counter medications/an elimination diet/physical therapy*) to relieve the symptom.

This has affected my ability to (*work/exercise/get out of bed/be outdoors/concentrate for long periods of time*).

Put together a timeline. Think about the onset of the problem(s) at hand. Which symptom(s) began first? Did they all begin simultaneously? Has one been a chronic problem for years that recently changed in frequency and/or intensity? Does one symptom exacerbate another?

204

Then consider anything from your medical history that might be relevant. If you have a compilation of your records (see page 125), flag anything that might be connected. Even if your provider already has access to this information, it's helpful to draw their attention to anything relevant up front so they don't have to search.

Once you have assembled all this information, you can craft your opening statement. For example:

Two months ago, I started having nerve pain in my upper neck following strenuous activity. The pain tends to last for seven to eight hours once it starts. I've tried Advil, applying heat, and chiropractic sessions every month, but nothing makes a difference. Because of the pain, I've had difficulty sleeping for the last several weeks. I used to get eight hours a night, but I'm now getting closer to four. The neck pain also gives me migraines, which are a new symptom for me and debilitating. I'm missing work and family activities because light and noise exacerbate the migraines. I have a history of disc problems and chronic lower-back pain. I had X-rays one year ago that ruled out certain causes, but they didn't come to any conclusions. The notes from this visit are here in my medi-cal record.

REALITIES ABOUT DIAGNOSIS

Three years ago the National Academy of Medicine reported that people are likely to receive a late or incorrect diagnosis at least once in their lives. That's twelve million people annually.[1] To complicate the picture, there are several types of diagnostic failings. Understanding these concepts from the outset, while you're receiving care, can help you guide discussions with your provider.

Among the different types of misdiagnosis are:

Misdiagnosis: The general term for the incorrect assessment and diagnosis of a disease.

Missed diagnosis: The failure to identify and diagnose a disease already under-way.

Delayed diagnosis: Failure to identify, diagnose, and intervene at the onset of symptoms, resulting in delayed care and poorer prognosis once the disease is diagnosed.

Overdiagnosis: An accurate diagnosis and intent to intervene for a disease that will not cause problems in the patient's

206

lifetime, such as a slow-growing cancer in an eighty-year-old patient.

Underdiagnosis: A condition or disease that goes undiagnosed within a specific population or context — for example, heart attacks in women or unaccompanied by pain.

How Providers Think

Confidence. It plays a critical role in how providers come to conclusions when they diagnose patients, and research now shows it's the thing most likely to get us into trouble.

One of the tenets of medical education is using a form of deductive reasoning to come to decisions about what is going on with a patient — what disease or condition is expressing itself, and how to proceed. Deductive reasoning, also called top-down reasoning, can take the form of decision-making trees. Imagine a hospital room where a medical student is being interrogated by the attending doctor at a bedside:

Attending: Please present on Mrs. Fisher.

Student: Mrs. Fisher is a forty-five-year-old female with lobular carcinoma in situ, admitted on 8/1 due to postsurgical complications. She has a progressive, two-day history of neutropenia and is intermittently febrile at

38.3°C. Source of infection remains unclear.
  Attending: What's your assessment?

What follows is a path down an algorithm tree that's been freshly etched into the medical student's brain. They'll come up with differentials, or, possible diagnoses based on symptoms, and either rule them out or hone in on them based on the case at hand.

Student: Based on A and B, we've ruled out C, D, and E. Because of F, it's likely to be in category G, so the possibilities are X and Y.

These decision-making trees are the scaffolding for making a diagnosis and executing a plan. Providers use them to create an accurate picture of their patient's symptoms and implement treatments accordingly.

But these trees can be inflexible. The provider often reproduces them for each patient displaying the same set of symptoms, and uses their pathways over and over again through experience. This model usually works, but it also has the tendency to place more emphasis on ticking off boxes than on thinking outside them, leading to diagnostic misses.

It can add up to a restrictive thought process that puts a provider on a path straight to *I'm so right, I'm wrong,* a path we've all traversed at some point or another.

The Science of Diagnosis

In order to understand the neural underpinnings of this medical tendency toward premature certainty, researchers at the University of São Paulo Medical School in Brazil used functional magnetic resonance imaging (MRIs) to examine how doctors' brains work as they make diagnoses.

In the study, primary care providers were shown a set of symptoms and asked to identify the disease they indicated. For example, a productive cough, sore throat, inflammation of the bronchioles, and chest tightness were linked to bronchitis. Interspersed throughout these identifications, the physicians were shown words and phrases and asked to name the animal they indicated — for example, the words "meow," "domestic animal," and "black fur" suggested a cat.

The researchers demonstrated that the areas of the brain that lit up during these processes were the same — naming a cat and using symptoms to diagnose a disease required the same cognitive pathways.

Next, the MRIs showed that when the physicians had to think about less-specific diagnostic information that could be associated with any number of diseases (nasal congestion, for instance), activity increased in the brain system known as the frontoparietal attention network — that is, their attention intensified. But the physician's attention was reduced if they were given highly specific information, strongly associated with a particular disease, at the start. This suggests that as a provider becomes more certain of a diagnosis, their attention to the matter decreases.

In other cases, symptoms or conditions that result from a different problem are dismissed or looped into the primary diagnosis. This was also shown in the São Paulo study: Physicians associated low thyroxine with hypothyroidism (which makes sense), but this interrupted any investigation of depression — which can appear with hypothyroidism and requires a separate course of action. If you're told an animal has whiskers, laps milk, purrs, and naps, you're likely to think: house cat! But what if it's one of those domesticated foxes?

Other studies have corroborated the São Paulo study. One showed that if, at the beginning of a medical encounter, providers are given a list of possible diagnoses that all merit equal consideration, they are more likely to make an accurate diagnosis. In essence, overcertainty and overconfidence early on in a clinical encounter increase the likelihood of premature diagnosis — a common source of medical error.

So what can you do about the possibility of diagnostic mistakes? Well, just knowing that it's a phenomenon will change the way you approach a medical encounter. It's a reminder that things are always a little more complicated than they seem, so don't be afraid to push back or ask a provider to explain their reasoning if they rush straight to what they think is a bulletproof conclusion but you're not convinced. You can also contribute ideas about what *you* think a problem might be, and doing so is likely to be more beneficial at the *beginning* of the encounter, and if you include more than one option.

Earlier, in "Should I Google My Symptoms?" in chapter 4, I outlined ways to use (and not use) the Internet as a tool to understand your symptoms and prepare to navigate the medical encounter. Later, in "Mastering Disease," there's more information about how to master this process, especially when you have a chronic illness. For now, though, just remember that providers' brains work in patterns, and pushing them to think in less rigid, self-contained ways, while acknowledging and utilizing their expertise, can elevate the quality of care you receive.

NINE:
NAVIGATING TOUCHY TERRITORY

PREVENTIVE CARE SCREENINGS
Stemming from a public-health effort to mitigate the impact of common diseases, all Marketplace health plans and most other insurance plans cover preventive screenings and services free of charge. This means no co-payment or coinsurance, whether or not you've met your deductible. The following sections will give you advice on what screenings to get, when.

Standard Recommendations
Knowing what preventive care screenings you need is unfortunately more complicated than simply following recommendations and showing up for appointments. Recommendations are inconsistent, namely for cancer screenings. For instance, the American Cancer Society (ACS) and the National Comprehensive Cancer Network (NCCN) put forth screening recommendations that

conflict with each other and with those of the US Preventive Services Task Force, on which Marketplace coverage for screenings is based. This means experts have weighed the evidence on prevention and come to different conclusions. To illustrate the magnitude of these inconsistencies, there is a ten-year age difference between when the ACS recommends women begin annual mammographies and when the US Preventive Services Task Force recommends that women begin biennial mammography. That's disconcerting news. Insurance coverage for screenings varies depending on which organization the insurance provider follows, so your cancer prevention care may be based on which insurance you have rather than your risk profile. It creates confusion for everyone.

In an effort to help patients handle these discrepancies, the Prevent Cancer Foundation has a digital tool that lists screening recommendations from all leading organizations. It also allows you to review insurance plans by state to find out what screenings your insurance covers. It can be found at http://www.preventcancer.org/education/cancer-screening-coverage. I recommend taking a look.

Determining Your Risk Profile

Decisions to get certain screenings shouldn't be based solely on any of the national recommendations. These matters are nuanced and merit a dedicated conversation with your care team, taking into account your unique risk profiles for specific diseases. And it's more complicated than genetics. Ninety to ninety-five percent of cell mutations that result in breast cancers, for instance, are not hereditary, meaning there are other salient risk factors to evaluate with your provider.

Some patients have an unusually high risk and should screen earlier and more frequently than what's typically recommended. Effective prevention also requires more than just a conversation about when and how often: Some screenings might be problematic for certain individuals, for example by leading to a cascade of unnecessary intervention if something turns up positive (see "Realities About Diagnosis," beginning on page 206). This is a controversy impacting older adults. As you can see, deciding when to get screened depends, and it's complicated.

Catching disease early rests on a partnership between you and your primary care provider. Make sure you're prepared when

214

you sit down with them to discuss your risk profile so your conversation is personalized and relevant. If you've done a little work on the front end to determine your inherent risk for, say, breast or ovarian cancer, the conversation with your provider can jump right to the preventive piece. There are excellent resources to help you assess your risk and put the wheels in motion for early detection. Getting your initial risk profile just requires spending a little time reading.

I direct friends and patients to http://www.assessyourrisk.org to help them get a solid handle on their risk of breast and ovarian cancer. Its bright, nonintimidating interface will walk you through a comprehensive, straightforward test that leads to a risk percentage. When you finish, you can read about the various factors working for and against you that determine your lifetime risk, and see what lifestyle factors you can modify. You can also email a PDF directly to yourself and your provider. The site also equips patients with contacts for top genetic counselors in every zip code, teaches women how to notice changes in their bodies, and outlines the latest risk-reduction options to discuss at appointments.

I also recommend http://screeningforlife .ca. The Canadian-based site has a straightforward, useful risk-profile test for overall cancer risks.

At your next appointment with your primary care provider, use the following questions to open a dialogue about your individual risk factors and which screenings you may need to adjust:

Based on my medical history and current state of health, do I fall in an exceptional risk category for any diseases or conditions?

What organization do you look to for screening recommendations?

What tests or screenings might I need to have earlier in life or more frequently?

If I do get this test or screening outside the standard recommendations, can you assist me in getting my insurance to cover it?

If you do decide you need specific prevention services, you may find that your insurance provider is merciless about coverage. (A list of the preventive services covered free of charge by Marketplace insurance plans can be found on page 567.) In that case, you will need to discuss your options with your provider and weigh the pros and cons of waiting to have the screening when it's covered, or paying out of pocket.

The message here: Effective prevention, especially for cancers, requires legwork to determine your personal risk and an open, ongoing conversation with your care team.

VACCINES

I want to make one thing crystal clear for the record — my research and the serious medical problems found in those children were not a hoax and there was no fraud whatsoever. Nor did I seek to profit from our findings. . . . Despite media reports to the contrary, the results of my research have been duplicated in five other countries. . . . Since the *Lancet* paper, I have lost my job, my career and my country. To claim that my motivation was profit is patently untrue. I will not be deterred — this issue is far too important.

— ANDREW WAKEFIELD, DISGRACED RESEARCHER ACCUSED OF FRAUD AND CONFLICT OF INTEREST AFTER HIS 1998 PAPER LINKED VACCINATION TO AUTISM

Those are the words of a disgraced man attempting to save his ass. Excuse my French, but if you knew the fallout Wakefield caused in the healthcare world (one from which we are still recovering, two decades later) you'd find even better French to use.

There is considerable rancor around vaccination. It's a topic fraught with history, toxic capitalism, and misinformation, with the result that many modern patients either adopt firm beliefs about vaccines or assume a neutral stance and approach them with a lackadaisical attitude.

However, if you delve into the medical literature, the information is clear and straightforward: Vaccines protect, and their benefits far outweigh their risks.

It's time for a final shift in collective attitude when it comes to vaccinating. Time we not only accept the truth about vaccines (their purpose, safety, and efficacy) but also reprioritize them at different stages of life.

I'll talk more about the benefits of vaccines in a moment, but for now suffice it to say that vaccines protect your health and the health of your community at large. They are essential not only during infancy (which is often when the most care and attention are devoted to following a vaccination schedule) but throughout life, including its latter chapters. It can be difficult for older adults to advocate for themselves and stay on an effective vaccination schedule, especially when their brief appointment time is taken up addressing other pressing issues. Help your parents just as you help your children, and prioritize your own immunity just as you would a baby's.

An Ode to the Flu Shot

Bring up vaccinations at a dinner party, and everyone seems to have an opinion. Bring up the flu shot, and people get downright militant.

"Haven't had one since childhood and" — knock on wood — "I *never* get sick."

"I got it and I still got the flu."

"I got the flu shot once and it actually *made* me get sick."

We are cavalier when it comes to the flu shot, and it's easy to understand why. On the one hand, the flu is horribly unpleasant. Work, leisure, and relaxation are lost to misery — to aches, chills, intractable nausea, and diarrhea in all their glory — sometimes for two to three weeks! On the other hand, a vaccination of any sort is invasive, and the flu shot is an annual inconvenience. Vaccines deliver a cocktail of viral strains to your system, which, when you're feeling fine, sounds like the stuff of science fiction.

I've waffled on this matter, and even skipped the shot a few years out of sheer laziness, but since becoming a nurse I've been of the staunch opinion that everyone over the age of six months should get an annual flu shot. If you are over the age of sixty, pregnant, or immunocompromised, it's especially ill-advised to skip it.

Every year, the flu shot changes. Its composition is determined not by a group of old docs sitting around a conference table at Walgreens but by a veritable United Nations of influenza. Organizations including the Centers for Disease Control and Prevention (CDC) in Atlanta, the Francis Crick Institute in London, and the National Institute of Infectious Diseases in Tokyo come together and pool data on the most prominent flu strains circling the globe each year. They collectively recommend vaccine combinations for the Northern and Southern Hemispheres, released in September and February, respectively. It's an inelegant and imperfect process — tracing a family of viruses constantly in flux is a difficult task — but it's diligent and informed, based on much more than capitalism. An effective vaccine isn't guaranteed — some years, recommendations are simply better than others. Nor is it guaranteed you won't get the flu even if you *do* get vaccinated, but the vaccine will soften a flu's intensity and duration.

The long-term impact of inflammation on the body is rarely discussed in regard to the flu, but the flu is the atomic bomb of inflammation. If you're young and healthy and you contract the flu, your recovery is almost a given. But the flu exposes you to weeks of inflammation, which in turn can increase your risk of disease later on, including stroke, heart attack, and certain cancers.

There is also the issue of herd immunity, the resistance to the spread of a disease in a given area when a majority of its inhabitants are vaccinated. The flu can be grave, literally and figuratively. It's estimated that thirty-six thousand people die from the flu every year in the United States. As I write this in the fall of 2018, one hundred children have already died from the flu this year. Some people don't receive the flu shot for reasons out of their control, such as a severe allergy,* a genetic condition, or a lack of resources. Those individuals rely on the rest of us to get vaccinated and protect our communities.

In summary, the benefits of the flu shot far outweigh the inconvenience. It's a sound defense against something considerably

* If you have an egg allergy, talk to your provider before getting a flu shot.

more unpleasant and costly than a poke and a sore deltoid. Get the shot when it comes on the market in early September (if you're in the Northern Hemisphere), on a day you're feeling well. Make an annual outing of it and follow it up with apple picking or a movie marathon.

VIRUSES AND BACTERIA

How incredible that microbes, invisible to the naked eye, have the power to wipe out entire civilizations. And that we've created antibiotics that have the power to stop infections that might otherwise stop us in our tracks. You can contract paratyphoid from a cream puff, and Azithromycin can save you. But these days, we down this miracle of modern medicine with the nonchalance of taking Advil, so when the day comes, it might not work!

Antibiotic Resistance

Bacteria are sophisticated, and they are smart. They create little solar systems on and in our bodies — outnumbering human cells ten to one! — without which we would perish. They are magical and terrible, and they can turn on us just as easily as they sustain us.

Superbugs, like the infamous MRSA

(methicillin-resistant Staphylococcus aureus), are the epitome of our relationship to bacteria gone awry, the outcome of a battle between nature and manmade solutions to survive it. At the end of the day, little microbes are still finding ways to outsmart us and our antibiotics.

For every million Staphylococcus aureus cells that an antibiotic kills, a few will stick around thanks to special mutations, superpowers they've developed to withstand the nuclear winter brought on by the antibiotic. Once these mutated bacteria begin to multiply, divide, and conquer, you have a new army of bacteria that can resist the antibiotic attacking them.

Penicillin and methicillin were used to treat staph infections starting in the 1950s, but then the staph bacteria mutated and became resistant. Today, 70 percent of healthcare workers are carriers of MRSA. The infection is so virulent, difficult to contain, and easily contagious that it's virtually everywhere. This process happens frequently. Macrolides, a class of antibiotics used to treat sexually transmitted infections (STIs) and respiratory infections, can become ineffective against a bacteria after only one mutation. The process takes just two mutations against quinolones, antibiotics used to treat bone and joint infections.

Is This Viral or Bacterial?

Most US antibiotic prescriptions are for respiratory symptoms, and research indicates that about half are unnecessary. In the winter, it's not that uncommon for patients to flock to clinics asking for antibiotics to treat the flu.

Remember this essential point when it comes to antibiotics: There are viral infections, and there are bacterial infections. *Antibiotics only work on the latter.*

So how do you know whether to go to the doctor or wait it out when you're down and full of phlegm? I can offer a few clues to help you know what you're dealing with and whether it's time to go in and be seen. But the only way to definitively determine whether something is viral or bacterial is usually through a lab culture, which takes approximately two days to produce results.

URI

Upper respiratory infections (URIs) are the most common conditions that bring patients in asking for antibiotics, yet more than half of these illnesses are viral in origin. The color of your secretions can give you insight: Viral infections usually produce **clear**

224

mucus, which gradually shifts to **yellow and green** as your body expends white blood cells to fight it off. **Rusty-red** sputum from coughs likely indicates a bacterial infection like pneumonia, or something more serious that requires medical attention straightaway.

Sore Throat

A handful of illnesses can affect the tonsils and cause a sore throat, and color can be instructive here as well. Use your phone's flashlight and take a good peer down there, or have someone help you out. White matter on the tonsils or throat can indicate a bacterial, viral, or fungal infection. The white spots can look like little veins or even cow spots and usually warrant a trip in to be seen, especially if accompanied with unremitting swelling and pain. Your provider may swab the area and complete a rapid-antigen detection test to see if the infection is indeed bacterial.

If an illness lingers for fourteen days, go see a provider. It's not unusual to get a secondary bacterial infection on top of a viral infection. This can happen in the sinuses, for example, when days of inflammation from a virus invite bacteria to join in on the fun. If you are prescribed an antiobiotic, ask your provider:

What are the side effects?

How likely is it that it will work for me again in the future if I take it now?

Would rest and fluids have a similar impact?

Can I wait a few days before I fill the prescription to see if the illness resolves?

Antibiotics

Below are some common types and examples of antibiotics, with instructions for their use. (Antibiotics of the same overall type can be recognized by the fact that they share a prefix or suffix.)

"Cef": cefdinir, cefixime

Never take these with alcohol (even just one drink), or you will experience an onset of flushing, sweating, heart pounding, and vomiting that will scare you off antibiotics for good. Don't worry, the pharmacist will remind you about this one.

"Cillin": amoxicillin, ampicillin, penicillin

Do not take these with food, as it

226

decreases absorption of medication.

"Cycline": doxycycline, tetracycline
Do not take these with antacids or aspirin, or if you're pregnant. Cover up from the sun while you're taking these and for five days following the last dose, as these antibiotics will cause you to burn more easily.

"Mycin": clindamycin, vancomycin
Can cause ringing in and damage to ears; alert your provider at any sign of this.

"Oxacin" or **"floxacin":** moxifloxacin, ofloxacin
Drink lots of water to avoid kidney stones. Cover up from the sun while you're taking these and for five days following the last dose, as these antibiotics will cause you to burn more easily. These antibiotics can also cause tendonitis — especially in older adults and people taking corticosteroids — so if you experience tendon pain, see your provider! In rare cases, these antibiotics can cause peripheral neuropathy (tingling, numbness, and burning in upper and lower extremities). If this happens, notify your provider.

"Sulf": sulfamethoxazole-trimethoprim, sulfasalazine

Drink lots of water to avoid kidney stones. Cover up from the sun while you're taking these and for five days following the last dose, as these antibiotics will cause you to burn more easily.

Suprainfections

Have you ever taken an antibiotic and wound up with a yeast infection or unremitting diarrhea? Antibiotics are effective, but they are also indiscriminate. Unable to tell the difference between good and bad bacteria, they kill everything in their wake, which means that the good guys who fend off infection from day to day become casualties.

Probiotics will help avoid this, but alert your provider if you notice any of the following signs that indicate your bacteria flora has been compromised and other microbes are taking advantage of the opportunity:

Itchy or furry tongue
Diarrhea
Vaginal or rectal itching

Should You Take the Full Course?

I won't pull you deep into the annals of medical history — suffice it to say that antibiotic resistance is a result of rampant antibiotic use over time. But it's medical dogma you're likely familiar with that patient adherence is partly to blame for this, and that you're to *always* take the full course *exactly* as prescribed through to the *last pill.* The rationale and accuracy of this theory is still up for debate in the field, however. Infectious disease experts Martin Llewelyn from the Brighton and Sussex Medical School and Tim Peto from the Oxford Biomedical Research Center in the *British Journal of Medicine* say "it is time for policymakers, educators and doctors to drop the 'complete the course' message and state that it is not based on evidence."[1] Their theory, supported by others in the field, is that the problem is not taking too few pills but taking too many.

According to the *Washington Post,* "Peto explained in an interview that as far as they could tell, the 'full course' idea originated with a speech in 1945 given by Nobel Prize winner Alexander Fleming. Fleming recounted a moving story involving a patient with a streptococcal throat infection who didn't take enough penicillin, and passed it on to his wife, leading to her death from the newly antibiotic-resistant strain." Their theory is that this incited a practice of telling patients to take every last pill even after feeling better, advice based on anecdotal, emotional evidence that doesn't have adequate research to support it, according to Peto.

As you're reeling from what are possibly decades of instructions from your provider to the contrary, the take-home message here is simple: Antibiotics are to be thought of as a precious resource and used only when absolutely necessary for the shortest amount of time possible. Check that your provider has prescribed the most conservative amount possible, and take as directed.

SEX

Let's briefly talk about sex. Not the birds and the bees, but the squirrelliness that comes with talking to a medical professional about who you're necking with. It's awkward for the majority, a reminder that for all our wild ways those puritanical forebears still have their bony hands clamped on our shoulders.

In your middle school sex-ed class that awkwardness might have led to a fit of giggles, but for adults it's transmuted to something that looks more like shame. Shame that leads to omission when someone in flowery scrubs looks you plainly in the face and asks about your sexual proclivities. But evasiveness can put you and others at risk. Our reasons for not wanting to talk about such things outnumber, but don't outweigh, the reasons we should talk about them.

Sex carries such personal and intimate freight that it's difficult to pull back and view it as a physical act that impacts health just like diet and exercise. For nurses and doctors, receiving information about your sex life is about as charged as reading your blood pressure. We don't judge it, and we're not remotely embarrassed by it. A good scrotal sling joke might make us laugh, but truthfully, we've seen it all. Thousands of genitals. Countless cases of STIs. These things don't faze us. We're simply collecting information about a piece of your life that, for our purposes, amounts to a swapping of cells that can plant disease (or another human) inside someone's body.

Here are a few tips for discussing your sex life with your provider.

Relevant Details
At routine appointments, you and your provider should discuss:

Your sexual health history

Your current number of sexual partners
Exposure to any new sexual partners in
  the last year
The sex of the person or people you're
  having sex with
Any symptoms that gave you pause, even
  if they came and went

There are many excellent resources available to support you in managing your sexual health — even if you are without insurance, or don't have a strong relationship with a primary care provider. Planned Parenthood is an expert source of information and education on sexual health, and it helps patients regardless of insurance. Its reputation precedes itself, so I won't say much here, except that you should use it and do what you can to support its existence.

Most urban settings also have clinics where one can get an STI test on short notice, either for free or for a nominal fee with a sliding scale. Using the website https://www.powertodecide.org/sexual -health/your-sexual-health/find-clinic, you can locate the center that's most convenient to you.

Sexually Transmitted Infections

Almost all urban areas have substantial rates of undetected sexually transmitted infections (STIs), especially of those that are silent and asymptomatic, like human papillomavirus (HPV). (See page 234 for a discussion on what's up with Gardasil.) Because there are cultural and historical stigmas around STIs, many people forgo routine screenings and avoid conversations with their providers about sexual health until something erupts below the belt.

This is not the beginning of a sex-ed course or a PSA, but rather a nudge to develop a rapport with your provider that allows for frank discussion about sexual health. Adolescents need cultural and parental support in initiating these discussions, and sexually active older adults (in whom STIs are on the rise) need to be on the ball about bringing up sex at appointments.

STIs might feel like a scarlet letter on a clean bill of health, and many patients, even after being diagnosed and treated, agonize unnecessarily and in silence because of misinformation and stigma. Remember, your medical providers are a source of support on any issues regarding STIs, and they can often allay your worst fears.

What's the Deal with HPV and Gardasil?

Gardasil is a safe vaccine that protects against some of the most dangerous strains of human papillomavirus (HPV), a sexually transmitted infection that's the culprit of health problems from genital warts to several types of cancer in people of both sexes. (And not only cervical cancer — HPV strains have been linked to mouth and throat cancers as well.)

Fortunately, Gardasil is extremely effective. Four years after the original vaccine was released, the prevalence of targeted HPV strains among female adolescents had decreased by 56 percent.[2]

Compared to, say, the chicken pox vaccine, Gardasil is relatively new, and it's been adopted more slowly because of persistent (and false) myths that getting the vaccine promotes adolescent promiscuity. Despite this noise, according to midwife Lucille Glick, vaccination rates are on the rise in the United States. Gardasil 9, the newest vaccine on the market, protects against more than double the number of HPV strains that the original vaccine did.[3]

We are still learning more about HPV in the healthcare community and continuing to provide patient education on the topic, but for now, appreciate the HPV vaccine's standing on the list of important immunizations to receive to prevent cancer secondary to a viral infection.

TRAUMA-INFORMED CARE

In the mid-nineties, the CDC and Kaiser Permanente discovered an exposure that dramatically increased the risk for seven out of ten of the leading causes of death in the United States. In high doses, it affects brain development, the immune system, hormonal systems, and even the way our DNA is read and transcribed. Folks who are exposed in very high doses have triple the lifetime risk of heart disease and lung cancer and a twenty-year difference in life expectancy. And yet, doctors today are not trained in routine screening or treatment. Now, the exposure I'm talking about is not a pesticide or a packaging chemical. It's childhood trauma.

— DR. NADINE BURKE HARRIS

Our understanding of trauma — as healthcare professionals, patients, and citizens — is evolving. It's a delicate word, and a concept that takes many shapes. In the healthcare system we see not only individual trauma but also cultural and historical trauma that impacts the health of populations and generations.

Trauma is a loaded word socially, but it has different meanings in the medical world. Blunt trauma. Traumatic brain injury. Trauma-informed care. The last is the one we're discussing here. In the mid-nineties, the chief of Kaiser Permanente's Department of Preventive Medicine, Dr. Vincent Felitti, teamed up with the CDC to undertake a landmark study that demonstrated a clear link between exposure to adversity in childhood and health problems later in life. Dr. Nadine Burke Harris, along with other experts, has resurrected and championed this research. The premise is that adverse childhood experiences (we call them ACEs) have a profound impact on brain development and bodily health, in childhood and later in life. We have only a nascent understanding of this correlation — it is a public health crisis we have yet to tackle.

The research can be distilled to this: If an individual experienced trauma in childhood, such as extreme abuse, neglect, or having a parent with a mental health condition or drinking problem, they possess a higher risk for a host of diseases due to inflammatory and neural processes set off by stress. This holds true regardless of affluence, zip code, and even modifiable lifestyle choices (such as smoking and drinking, which might be used as coping mechanisms).

This occurs because at the cellular level, when a child is in fight-or-flight mode (frightened, hypervigilant, with a racing heart) a cascade of stress hormones floods the body and alters specific circuits in the brain. As this cascade occurs repeatedly over time during critical periods of development, it alters neuroarchitecture, and it results in alterations of immunity, hormonal regulation, and overall systemic health.

Assessment for trauma of this nature is slowly becoming a standard of care, and providers are asking new questions to screen for it. Where we once referred patients to mental health or social services, we now see these issues as tied to the physiological, and ultimately under the umbrella of medical care. We are learning to be more sensitive to a patient's trauma history in triggering settings, such as ERs, and we are incorporating prevention of trauma-related diseases into our practices.

The medical encounter should provide an opportunity for the patient to talk about past and present stressors. If you are among the 67 percent of people who have experienced trauma — or experiences it actively

— it's important to bring it up with your primary care provider, and therefore essential to find one you feel comfortable doing so with.

If you need help initiating this conversation, you can start by completing the ACE evaluation and bringing it to your PCP. You do not have to get into the nature of your trauma, or anticipate a Freudian analysis; however, for health reasons it's an important topic to address. This way, they can manage the risks it's introduced to your overall health and support you in establishing resilience. The ACE questionnaire can be found at https://www.ncjfcj.org/sites/default/files/Finding%20Your%20ACE%20Score.pdf.

MYTHS ABOUT WEIGHT AND HEALTH

As a country and a medical community, we place too much emphasis on weight as an indicator of health. It's convenient to blame obesity for everything wrong with Americans' health: It places the onus for change on the patient, and it fits easily into a culture where fat shaming is embedded in the things we consume. It's true that obesity and metabolic syndrome are serious health conditions, but they are the extreme end of the story. They are not most people. Outside these categories, it's often more dangerous to one's health to be five pounds under-weight than to be what we consider over-weight based on body mass index (BMI). A 2016 study with a sample of more than 5,400 adults found that half of overweight people and one-third of obese people are "metabolically healthy." That means despite their excess pounds, many overweight and obese adults have healthy levels of good cholesterol, blood pressure, blood glucose, and other risks for heart disease.[4]

The misleading messages about weight that the medical world sends on full blast are dangerous to patients. It's already uncomfortable to get on the scale, but add-ing the dread of a slap on the wrist or a talking-to because you've put on weight is a reason many people avoid routine care. It's dangerous and counterintuitive for provid-ers to insist that being overweight, even slightly, is an extreme health risk. It ignores evidence that suggests weight isn't that important if other aspects of a healthy life-style are in place.

If you are afraid to go to the doctor because you don't want to step on the scale, that's valid. But don't let a broken cultural attitude prevent you from getting care. If your PCP harps on your weight at the expense of learning anything else about your lifestyle habits (the way you handle stress, or your eating habits), it would be good to question their thinking, or find someone new.

TEN:
HOW TO AVOID A
WILD-GOOSE CHASE

In this section, you'll find a few of the most prevalent afflictions — IBS, headaches, and back pain — that bring patients into the healthcare system looking for relief. These ailments also have the potential to send you on a wild-goose chase, exposing you to risk and expense along the way.

You can always push these matters ahead full steam. Depending on the severity of your issue, you may be ready to do everything and anything possible to determine its cause and find a solution. If, on the other hand, you're in the early steps of getting assessments for these conditions, or deciding whether to be seen for them, below are things to consider.

IRRITABLE BOWEL SYNDROME
Does anyone have any dietary restrictions?

Yes. Your friend is avoiding red meat. Her partner is off nightshades. Mom has announced she's going gluten-free this holiday season (or, as my ninety-four-year-old grandmother calls it, "glutton-free").

More often than not, the catalyst for these radical acts of deprivation is gastrointestinal distress. When the medical community can't determine its cause, they call it irritable bowel syndrome (IBS). What a term! It's vague, given the vast, complex abyss of our gastrointestinal (GI) system — if you need a refresher, just watch an episode of *The Magic School Bus.* It's also an understatement for a condition of the bowels that can be as raging as a Spanish bull.

IBS is one of the most common functional GI disorders worldwide, affecting approximately 15 percent of the population and accounting for 3.5 million annual provider visits. It's categorized as a "functional" disease because it's defined by its symptoms, rather than an identifiable underlying cause. You probably know someone who's struggled with it, or you yourself have abandoned your cart in the middle of a Costco trip in a violent dash for the nearest bathroom.

Amid those 3.5 million visits for IBS-related symptoms are countless incidents of patients being exposed to risky tests and sent off for unnecessary surgeries. Recent studies have shown that patients (mostly women) are five times more likely to be misdiagnosed in response to seeking treatment for what is in fact IBS than for other ailments. The outcome can be as extreme as intra-or extra-abdominal surgeries (cholecystectomy, appendectomy, or hysterectomy — removal of the gallbladder, appendix, or uterus). Even if things don't go south and result in an -ectomy (the removal of an organ), there's also the problem and expense of unnecessary procedures — who wants a colonoscopy or radiation exposure if it isn't warranted?

If you think you may suffer from IBS and are considering medical treatment, arm yourself with the following information:

- IBS (irritable bowel syndrome) and IBD (inflammatory bowel disease) are distinctly different maladies, though they both inflict GI discomfort. Inflammatory bowel diseases have organic correlates — meaning distinct biological causes, such as ulcers along the inside of the intestine — and are easier to diagnose. If there is blood, mucus, or something that looks like coffee grounds in your stool, and/ or if you've experienced weight loss that coincides with symptom onset, definitely go see your provider.

- With IBS, it's better to start with your own interventions before crossing over into the healthcare world. Lifestyle changes you can take include decreasing caffeine, limiting your alcohol consumption, and altering your diet in different ways. Take time to implement them and assess their effect before moving on to the next steps.
- Many patients end up at a GI specialist for testing, simply to be sent off with a little pamphlet about the FODMAP diet. This is becoming standard practice, as the diet has demonstrated success across the board in minimizing symptoms. Rather than beginning with an appointment, try the FODMAP diet first. It can be found here: https://www.monashfodmap.com/i-have-ibs/starting-the-low-fodmap-diet/.
- If your symptoms are severe and distressing enough that you would like to begin with or move toward medical intervention, plan for your communication with your provider. Make a list of patterns and what you eat (using pen and paper or a symptom tracker app) over the two weeks leading up to

your appointment. Be very specific about symptoms, onset, duration, alleviating factors, and lifestyle patterns that aggravate the symptoms. This way, you'll have data to present and won't wind up in a specialist's office with little to say besides "cramps, diarrhea, or constipation" when they are trying to get to the bottom (!) of a disease that could be anything.

HEADACHES

Headaches can also open up a Pandora's box of unnecessary interventions. If you're experiencing frequent headaches, try lifestyle modifications first. Altering your sleep habits or diet, managing stress, and trying over-the-counter pain medications are all good first steps for the majority of headaches caused by tension. If these don't help, see a provider for a physical examination.

Because a headache's source can be hard to pin down for even the best specialists, an MRI or CT scan can seem like the most logical next step. These imaging tests, however, rarely yield anything conclusive. The only certainties are that they're expensive, and they expose you to radiation. If a provider recommends having one done and provides a good rationale, or a physical reveals any of the below symptoms, these are occasions to proceed with imaging:

Abnormal reflexes
Weakness on one side of the face or body
Unsteady gait
Double vision
Vision loss
Abnormalities of the pupils
Confusion

Below are also headache situations in which you should seek immediate treatment, and a scan is warranted:

Headaches that are sudden or feel like something is bursting inside your head.
Headaches that are different from other headaches you've had, especially if you are age fifty or older.
New headaches in a person with cancer
Headaches in immunosuppressed people
Persistent headaches after a head injury
Persistent fever
No response to treatment
Headaches that happen after you have been physically active.
Headaches with other serious symptoms, such as a loss of control, a seizure or fit,

or a change in speech or alertness.*

LOWER BACK PAIN

Most people with lower back pain feel better in about a month, whether they get an imaging test or not. Imaging tests here can also lead to additional procedures that complicate recovery. One large study of people with back pain found that those who had imaging tests soon after they reported the problem fared no better, and sometimes did worse, than people who took simple steps like applying heat, staying active, and taking over-the-counter (OTC) pain relievers. Another study found that back-pain sufferers who had an MRI in the first month were eight times more likely to have surgery, but they didn't recover faster.

In some situations, it does make sense to get an MRI. These include:

History of cancer
Unexplained weight loss
Fever
Recent infection

* Adapted from the Choosing Wisely Patient Resource Campaign, http://www.choosingwisely.org/patient-resources/imaging-tests-for-head aches/.

Loss of bowel or bladder control
Abnormal reflexes
Loss of muscle power or feeling in the legs

Otherwise, try using a heating pad, staying active, sleeping with a pillow between or underneath your knees, physical therapy, and/or OTC pain relievers like ibuprofen.

■ ■ ■ ■

PART IV
WHEN IT'S CHRONIC:
NAVIGATING
LONG-TERM AND
ONGOING MEDICAL
PROBLEMS

■ ■ ■ ■

Many patients say that managing a chronic illness feels like having another job — one that renders you familiar with the world of modern medicines, or at least its powers, laws, and roadblocks.

It's likely that if you fall into this category, you've developed your own repertoire to make the whole operation run more smoothly. Topics in the following section include how to pull the most relevant research on your condition, essential practices for coordinating your care between offices and specialists, addressing chronic pain, and asserting your priorities. It also provides resources for educating friends and family and strengthening your support network.

Eleven:
Brewing Problems

Some health issues have a sudden onset and a relatively short half-life. Others are more of a chronic brew. Symptoms gradually surface, or wax and wane in intensity. Sometimes a symptom on its own is enough to alarm you and send you to your provider. Other times, seemingly unrelated symptoms come in tandem or one after another in quick succession, causing you to wonder if the numbness and tingling is a symptom of the disease you're already medicating, a side effect of that medication, or an unrelated issue entirely.

Times when new symptoms manifest in the body can be emotionally trying. Vulnerability and distress intensify when we don't know the source of the pain, the symptom, or the side effect. Turning to medical experts for guidance and assessment can feel both urgent and daunting, especially when there's such limited time to give them insight into your physical reality.

The modern medical system doesn't always deal with these brewing problems well: It's stingy with its time, specialists often fail to coordinate with one another, and there's a widespread tendency to slap a diagnosis on a patient too quickly. Alternately, there are times an accurate diagnosis can take years; countless scans, tests, or episodes disseminated through space and time. For this reason patients with chronic illness spend significantly more on medical care as providers try to rule out diseases and use trial and error with medications.

The following sections are structured to support you as you attempt to get a diagnosis. They'll also empower you to trust yourself and elicit support from several resources as you wait for one.

SPECIALISTS AND REFERRALS

Our culture has an obsession with specialists. Patients and providers alike have a particular affinity for them: providers, because they can punt off a case that eludes them or that they don't have sufficient time to get to the root of; patients, because they assume a referral means they're finally being heard and that they've been granted access to someone who can help. But while specialists are vital to the healthcare system and they indeed help many of us, they're not always the answer. The vantage point of a specialist is often limiting — they're not trained, like an internist or a family medicine provider is, to hone in on the interrelationships of the body's systems. They assess an illness through a specific lens, limited by the nature of their specialty.

Keep the following in mind when you consider entering this territory looking for a diagnosis.

"Prescribe and Refer"

A pattern called "prescribe and refer" gets at the heart of the problem with our proliferation of specialist send-offs. It works like this:

You present to your primary practitioner with a cluster of symptoms you're experiencing.

The provider runs a battery of tests. If they don't arrive at a clear-cut diagnosis, they may move on to treating the symptoms with medication. They may toss around words like "functional" or "idiopathic" at this point — meaning they do not have an answer.

If the problem does not resolve from treating the symptoms alone, the provider refers you to a specialist. The entire process then stands to be repeated if things do not resolve.

The specialist may send you to a different specialist, or ask you about psychiatric symptoms — like depression or anxiety — that would confirm it's psychosomatic (relating to mental health).

Of course this doesn't happen 100 percent of the time; specialists are vital, but it's a pervasive practice. It's also a significant source of disappointment, frustration, stress, and financial investment for patients. On this topic, the experts I interviewed said the same thing: Be wary when this bouncing-around-to-specialists commences, because this is where the role of overseeing the whole case and connecting the dots is often abandoned. There's no one putting the puzzle together or ensuring that clues are shared and discussed between providers. (Page 276 will cover this issue of care coordination extensively.) Often the answer is there, in the picture as a whole including specialist input, but no one steps up to put all the pieces together.

But you can disrupt this ineffective pattern and fare better as you move through the specialist train. Once the medical web extends from your PCP's office and includes different specialists, you simply hold down the fort, knowing you are the single most important conduit of information

Maximizing Specialist Appointments

At each specialist appointment, ask that they do a full physical assessment themselves. Don't let them jump to talking about prescriptions, quick surgical fixes, or referrals without so much as examining you.

It's likely that a waiting game will follow your initial appointment, and this is where things get slippery. The provider may say they need to order tests or send you to another specialist, or they may hint at a rather amorphous plan that involves a combination of treating symptoms and waiting and seeing.

Before the appointment concludes, get answers to the following questions so you are not lost in the abyss.

If tests are ordered:

What are the specific tests, and what are they for?
When will they be scheduled?

When will you have the results?

How will the results be communicated to you?

If medication is prescribed:

Is it to treat the symptoms, or a disease?

What are the side effects?

Will you need to stay on them indefinitely?

If you get a referral:

Why does the provider recommend this particular specialist?

Will specialist A remain involved in your care?

Before you leave, know the specifics of the game plan. What are you waiting on before the next appointment — a test result? A referral? A trial of a new medication to see how it helps?

The bottom line: Go in, present your case in a thoughtful and articulate way, and focus on care coordination. Don't assume there's a greater plan you're not privy to, but instead leave with a clear sense of the plan and a timeline for next steps. If trips to specialists don't yield any answers, take the notes and results back to your PCP and go over them together.

WHEN YOU CAN'T GET A DIAGNOSIS

Sometimes not having a diagnosis is worse than having a bleak one. The medical world relies on diagnoses to guide treatment, insurance companies demand them if they're to pay, and patients look to them for validation that what they're experiencing is real.

Struggling with debilitating symptoms without a diagnosis can bring on its own kind of hell. Like the nightmare where you're yelling out for help and no one can hear you, or nothing comes out of your mouth when you try to speak. Or the one where you've been framed and not a soul in the village, not even your own mother, believes in your innocence.

When you can't get a diagnosis, frustration often results from dealing with a medical team operating on trial and error, offering only small bouts of remission or alleviation. It's also isolating. There's a shared social understanding about cancer and ALS, but there's no real equivalent for chronic fatigue, or bouts of vertigo. There's a hierarchy of disease in our world, and when you don't have a label to put on your condition, there's extra strain in asking for accommodation and understanding from the people and institutions around us.

It can all add up to the worst of conclusions: *Am I imagining this?* This question logically follows the experience of being dismissed as an unreliable witness to the things going on inside you.

To find yourself somewhere in between suffering and treatment, without a light at the end of the tunnel, is a time of particular vulnerability. It's also a crucial point of decision-making, because you can either accept the question mark or tap into your reserves and keep trying to get an answer. As I say in this book's preface, this work can be exhausting and overwhelming when your stamina and health are compromised at the outset. While coordinating your specialty care is especially important here, it will also serve you to effectively communicate your pain, and enlist the support of your family and larger community. Here are additional tools and ideas.

TWELVE:
A FIELD GUIDE FOR PAIN

DESCRIBING PAIN

Pain is full of dichotomies. It is a human experience so unmistakable that to witness someone else in anguish transcends the need for communication. And yet when we're sitting in a clinician's office, pain is good at reminding us of the limits of language.

However it manifests, pain is the most common catalyst for excursions into the world of medicine. It sends us out for help.

Learn how to describe your pain. In most encounters, a numeric one-to-ten rating scale will be used to ask you about the severity of what you're experiencing. It's universally effective, but if you don't like working with it you can request another type of scale to communicate. There is a scale showing faces in pain, as well as other visual analogue scales. In the following pages you'll find the language and ideas to help you discuss pain in more dynamic terms, which will benefit you as well when talking to your providers.

Describe the Logistics of the Pain

When did the pain begin?
What is the pain's duration?
What relieves the pain?
What aggravates it?

Words to Describe Pain

Sharp
Shooting
Tender
Burning
Aching
Stabbing
Dull
Throbbing
Intense
Intermittent
Unrelenting

Effects of Pain

Does the pain cause changes in:

Respiration?
Heart rate?

Does the pain cause you to:

Blush?
Have a sudden muscular contraction?
Perspire?
Clench your teeth?

Impact on Your Life

Does the pain cause you to:

Withdraw from others?
Avoid activities?
Let go of personal hygiene?
Lose sleep?

USING NARRATIVE TO
COMMUNICATE ABOUT PAIN

Growing up includes the realization that a steadily increasing number of people you know have medical problems. For me it happened within a few years in my late twenties: One friend was diagnosed with MS, another with lymphoma; another called from across the world to tell me she had an ovarian tumor. The average healthy young person often lacks a framework to conceive of these real, life-impacting medical problems. I've been one of these lucky healthy people for the most part, and while being a nurse plants the reality of disease in front of me, I still struggle to understand the true impact of chronic pain or debilitating illness on someone's life. But I have learned lessons from being adjacent to suffering, both that of patients and of people close to me.

One lesson is that the prospect of relaying information or updating others on "how things are going" can be a daunting prospect for people struggling with chronic pain and illness. It requires one to construct a narrative while the story is still developing, or still eludes the patient themselves. And telling this story sometimes means relaying things that are too complicated to unpack in a period of time deemed socially acceptable when a friend or acquaintance asks how you're doing. Assembling the pieces of this story for providers as the clock is ticking in an exam room can also be a seemingly impossible task. And yet, as a nurse, I know how imperative it is for them to get this information.

It is vital for medical providers not only to hear but also to help create their patients' narratives. Friends and family can benefit from hearing the story of someone's pain because it elicits empathy, compassion, and support. But providers need to hear and understand these narratives for one explicit reason: to accurately understand the impact of pain or illness on quality of life and prioritize it accordingly.

There's very little in our medical system that supports being this vulnerable around a medical provider when appointments are increasingly rushed. When patients are in this position, their capacity is also often limited. Relaying a narrative can take significant mental and emotional reserves.

Tools are emerging to support patients through this process. Narrative medicine, a practice that began at Columbia University in New York, trains providers to create space in appointments for the narrative to emerge, and gives them tools to use it to direct the care they deliver. Today, programs around the country are beginning to adopt the practice.

Here is the concept as Columbia defines it:

The care of the sick unfolds in stories. The effective practice of healthcare requires the ability to recognize, absorb, interpret, and act on the stories and plights of others. Medicine practiced with narrative competence is a model for humane and effective medical practice. It addresses the need of patients and caregivers to voice their experience, to be heard and to be valued, and it acknowledges the power of narrative to change the way care is given and received.

For patients struggling with chronic illness, it's helpful to find providers, clinics, and hospitals that have training in narrative medicine. I recommend contacting Columbia directly and asking for patient resources (http://www.narrativemedicine.org). It may be too much to take on now, or at specific points in your disease, but it's a positive, evolving resource that many patients benefit from.

Pain Management in an Opioid Epidemic

Imagine a prominent scientist giving a talk on the opioid epidemic at a highly prestigious university. They stand at the podium in an auditorium endowed by and named after the Sackler family — whose patriarch made his fortune by introducing synthetic opioids to the US market. The stuff of a tragicomedy, it's surely happened on more than one occasion.

America is in the midst of a twenty-year public health crisis that can be traced to 1995, when Richard Sackler started Purdue Pharma and the company introduced OxyContin to the US market. It's estimated that the family has seen double digit billions in revenue from this pill, which was marketed to prescribers and patients as "the pain pill to start with and to stay with." In a story with classic strokes of greed and ego, the company was selective about the research it published and what its sales reps told the medical community.

By 2001, OxyContin had saturated the market. Meanwhile, and not coincidentally, pain management became a top priority in the healthcare industry. The Joint Commission, which accredits and certifies healthcare organizations, declared a veritable war on pain. They elevated it to a fifth vital sign, claiming that clinicians needed to be more proactive about addressing pain and staying on top of it at every turn. The result was a substantial shift in prescribing culture, which trickled downstream to impact the way pharmacies dispensed pain meds and the way pain management was taught in medical school. *Opioids are exceptionally effective in controlling pain, and when given in a controlled setting they aren't addictive. This is a miracle of modern medicine,* went the tune. *Extended release? Even better! Patients can take fewer pills.*

Moving ahead to today:

- If you use opioids for thirty days consecutively, there's a 50 percent chance you will still be using them in three years.
- Roughly one in three patients prescribed opioids for chronic pain misuses them.
- Between 8 and 12 percent of individuals who use opioids develop an opioid-use disorder.
- About 80 percent of people who use heroin first misused prescription opioids.

I was discussing these issues with my friend Jules recently, who, after tearing a tendon in his knee last fall, was handed a prescription for oxycodone with a number of refills that came to something like four hundred pills. Skeptical, and already dealing with various health problems that got in the way, he never filled the prescription.

"Well," I said, "they used to tell med students it wasn't addictive!"

"It's opium, it's the poppy!" he responded. "We've known forever that the poppy is trouble. I don't buy it."

We concluded that it's a classic American story. We discussed how he would never have been handed that prescription if he was less educated, or was of lower socioeconomic status, or wasn't a white man. Some patients in Jules' position would be denied the prescription; others would use it without a thought — and potentially greet a lifelong addiction.

There are four general contexts in which opioids are prescribed:*

When pain is acute and must be managed in the hospital (primarily procedure-related and postsurgical pain).

When an individual has little to no quality of life due to unmanaged pain (the pain is so unbearable the patient cannot resume multiple activities of daily life, such as bathing, dressing, or eating).

When a patient is at the end of life, and palliative (comfort) care is the focus.

On a short-term basis, following a procedure where the majority of recovery is done outside of the hospital.

* Opioids are prescribed outside these parameters as well. In these instances, the risk/benefit analysis comes down to the individual.

In addressing chronic pain, patients fall along a spectrum. There are those like Jules who, aware of the addictive potential of opioids, avoid using them under most circumstances. There are patients who use them and never develop abuse or addiction (the majority). There are patients who become addicted and start to doctor shop.

There are also, unfortunately, patients who struggle greatly with chronic pain that's inadequately managed as a result of the new shift in prescribing culture. Today, the directors of the National Institutes of Health and the National Institute on Drug Abuse say the public should no longer expect that chronic pain will be managed 100 percent by medications. Rather, they should expect pain to be managed enough so that they can maintain a quality of life. The directors encourage integrated approaches to pain, focusing on meditation, massage, and acupuncture as adjuncts to pharmacotherapy. Is yoga going to help someone with severe neuropathy? Maybe, maybe not. But the opioid epidemic means that patients have to build trust and open communication with providers so that pain is managed from a place of understanding rather than liability.

Until we can develop a drug that relieves pain as effectively as opioids but doesn't have their potential for abuse, patients must acknowledge and accept the ramifications of widespread opioid abuse. This understanding is essential to navigating pain management in the midst of an opioid epidemic.

If you do take opioids (and they can be an effective therapeutic option for many patients), here's what to know about taking them safely:

Don't abruptly stop taking them.

Don't take more than directed.

Never take them from another person (who has them left over from their wisdom teeth removal or back surgery, for example).

Don't store them in another bottle (e.g., an Advil bottle), as this puts others in your household at risk. One dose of methadone for an adult male can cause a child to die from respiratory arrest.

Keep them locked or on your person, out of reach of children and adolescents. Adolescents are the age group most likely to abuse this class of drugs.

Take the smallest effective dose, for the shortest amount of time possible.

Keep in close contact with a provider if you're taking them at home.

The appendix "Opioid Types and Side Effects" contains information on uncomfortable to fatal opioid side effects. It also lists generic and trade names of all opioids in use today so you can easily identify them.

Other Pain Management Options

Severe pain is usually managed, even in hospital settings, with a combination of drugs: an opioid plus a nonopioid (acetaminophen or ibuprofen). Studies have found that when groups of postoperative patients in a blind trial received a combination of either 1) Tylenol plus ibuprofen or 2) Tylenol plus an opioid, there was no clinical or statistical difference in pain management. Do with this information what you will! It's powerful.

This epidemic, like any, is categorized by its extremes. Most providers will listen to you, take your pain seriously, and help you resolve it. Most patients will not become addicted. But there are patients who don't receive the pain management they need, those who struggle with lifelong dependency, and those who die from misusing this extremely potent class of drugs. For this reason, providers and patients — unlike the Sacklers — must approach this topic with respect.

THIRTEEN:
MASTERING DISEASE

Read, learn, work it up, go to the literature.
Information is control.

— JOAN DIDION,
THE YEAR OF MAGICAL THINKING

WADING INTO THE LITERATURE

When you're navigating a chronic illness, a host of resources outside your provider's office can help you stay on top of research-based practice. There is an art to searching for medical information — one that, luckily, you have access to for free and don't have to tackle alone! Pair up with a librarian at a public or university library, or at the medical center where you're a patient. As a general principle, we would all fare better if we elevated librarians to a place of higher standing in our society. Their expertise extends far beyond cataloging. In an age where new information swirls around us at an inhuman pace, the ability to find what one is looking for is an art — one that librarians have mastered, including by searching the web. Rather than going it alone, Googling "Newest treatments for progressive-relapsing multiple sclerosis," and sifting through hundreds of thousands of results, find a librarian. Discuss your most pressing questions with them, and let them guide you through a search in their databases.

If you do want to do some research on your own, the National Library of Medicine is the place to start, as outlined in the section "Your Smartphone as a Medical Device." When you're searching the literature, look for "peer-reviewed research," "patient-centered outcome research," and "comparative effectiveness research." The terms indicate excellent methodological practices. Acquaint yourself with the nearest academic or teaching hospital (those nested within university settings in major cities). They tend to house specialists across disciplines, who are likely to approach your disease from many angles. They also house the most sophisticated medical libraries, with access to newly published studies the moment they become available. A comprehensive list can be found at http://www.aahcdc.org/about/members.

Once you've selected a university, locate the "research" section and browse the various departments and centers. On these pages, you can identify labs investigating topics related to your disease. These pages will allow you to find researchers (also called PIs, or principal investigators) considered experts in their areas, and browse their recent publications. It's common for researchers to list their academic email addresses on these sites, and if you have a specific question, you can reach out. While it's not part of their job description, I don't know a medical scientist around who wouldn't be willing to talk to a patient who approached them with a spirit of inquiry.

My instinct is to turn to the literature and immerse myself in facts when I'm overwhelmed by the unknown, but I appreciate that this isn't soothing or helpful to everyone. Still, your provider doesn't have the time or resources to familiarize themselves with every study or novel treatment option that springs up regarding your disease. Being able to do research yourself will help you advocate for yourself more effectively.

CLINICAL TRIALS

Clinical trials provide a portal to the expansive world of medical research. They grant access to medications, therapies, and sometimes life-prolonging procedures the mortal world of hospitals and practitioners don't yet have in their arsenal.

Clinical trials run the gamut, from providing a procedure at a reduced cost when your insurance won't cover it, to offering novel interventions. The latter don't come without risk, but if they're successful they may offer a great restoration of health and quality of life.

If you find yourself facing roadblocks at every turn — or even if you're just curious and would like to participate in research, a virtue in its own right — take a look at the current National Institutes of Health listings at http://clinicaltrials.gov. Here you'll find a registry and database of federally and privately supported clinical trials conducted in the United States and around the world. You can search at random for trials or look them up based on specific conditions, like multiple sclerosis or Parkinson's disease.

Research Match (http://www.research match.org) is a new tool that pairs you with studies based on your personal profile and medical history, whether you're healthy or struggling with a condition. The site provides a free, secure registry connecting you with researchers around the world who are looking for new participants or who specialize in areas of medicine you're looking for help in.

HOW TO BE A CONDUIT

Hermes has always been among my favorite characters in Greek mythology. He's an endearingly mischievous and compassionate god who liaises between worlds with the agility of a falcon and the charm of a politician. He's a messenger, and he takes great pride in his talent for protecting and relaying information.

Like Hermes is for the cosmos, you are a vital conduit of information in the world of modern medicine. In this world there's no herald, no spool of thread that connects the dots from one encounter to the next, no assurance that the parties involved in your care will get the message.

The unraveling of communication in a medical landscape is perhaps the single largest source of error. There are so many places and ways information can fall through the cracks — from building to building, PCP to specialist, and one appointment to the next.

It can be helpful to draw a web to understand the complexity of care coordination (like they have students do in nursing and medical school). Think of a person with a chronic illness and then list every person and entity that interfaces with their care in a given month. For example: primary care, specialist 1, specialist 2, pharmacist, mental health provider, laboratory, hospital, outpatient clinic, informal caregiver, advocate, social worker, physical therapist, nurse, insurance company.

Consider all the people orchestrating different elements of care, all the people between whom information essential to your case is passed back and forth after it's altered or updated. The abundant opportunities for dropping the ball become clear. It's a symphony without a conductor.

And this problem doesn't just apply to someone with a complex chronic illness.

Let's say you've been experiencing random bouts of numbness and tingling in your limbs, and it's alarming you. You present to your PCP, who decides to run some labs, which are collected by a medical aide and sent off. The results are processed in a few days. This part of the process is generally pretty streamlined.

When the results come back, someone in the office calls you, or you get a message via your online portal, to say that the labs came back normal. The PCP then decides to send you to a neurologist, who orders an MRI and another battery of tests, neither of which concludes much of anything. Then you're sent to an endocrinologist, and so on . . .

But who is making sure the tests ran by Provider A are reviewed by Provider B? Who is ensuring that your medical history has gotten more than a glance by each party? If Specialist A tells you to wait and monitor for other symptoms that could indicate X, who ensures that your PCP is aware and also monitoring you for X?

Rather than bouncing from one appointment to another, assuming everyone is talking behind the scenes and coordinating things, you have to channel Hermes. You have to know and protect the details of your case and ensure they get from place to place, person to person.

In order to coordinate your care, first you need an understanding of the basics of the plan. It's common for a patient's ears to perk up when they hear a specific diagnosis, or to selectively remember only the information that alarmed or relieved them and not process the rest. Providers are quick to walk out the door without explicitly describing the plan, because now patients are handed "recap" paperwork when they leave. These forms can be bare-bones and insufficient.

Your task here requires a back-and-forth with your provider until you understand what the follow-up plan will entail, to the extent that you can repeat it back to them.

Begin each appointment with a quick sentence or two that covers the plan, and where you are along the plan's trajectory. For instance:

Two weeks ago I saw Dr. Sharp for numbness and tingling in my lower legs, which began in June and occurs daily. She ordered these tests and sent me for an MRI, and now I'm here. She explained that possible diagnoses could be A, B, or C, so now I'm seeing you to determine or rule out MS.

Know your medical history and make a point of revisiting it with each provider. Don't assume that your PCP called the specialist to talk about your case. Don't assume the specialist was meticulously reading over your chart for an hour before they walked into the exam room. These things can happen, and should, but all too often they don't. For this reason, if your PCP intends to refer you to a specialist, it's worth asking them to call the specialist and discuss your case before sending you.

It might also be worthwhile to bring with you that compilation of your medical records (see page 125, "Your Medical Records"), or at least your healthbook, so you can easily reference appointment dates, provider names, tests, results, and other important details while the specialist is in the room with you. What constitutes important? Any serious conditions, surgeries, or symptoms you've had in the past. Any areas of concern in your family history. Abnormal test results of any sort from the last year, as well as your most recent test results. A list of any medications you've recently been prescribed.

Ensuring that your care is coordinated is a task that shouldn't fall on you, but it does. It's an imperative task that no one in the medical world is responsible for, and in its absence you will notice problems arising from information not dispersing where it needs to. Adopting this mind-set alone will greatly impact your care for the better.

PEER SUPPORT

Early into my relationship with my friend Gabe, I noticed that as we settled down at a bar or restaurant he would shuffle people around so he could sit at the end of the booth. It was a curious habit, an idiosyncrasy for someone who tends to drift around with ease.

A month or so into this game of musical

chairs, Gabe told me about his hearing. For several months he'd been experiencing intermittent deafness caused by a discordant, shrill ringing in his ears. The symptom appeared out of thin air, making the jump from unpleasant to painful in a fairly short amount of time.

As the winter progressed, other symptoms joined his ears in causing trouble. The most notable was spells of vertigo. He'd be dressed to head out to play basketball or at work, and suddenly be consumed by a bout of dizziness and nausea. He'd lose his balance and sense of corporeal perception, and experience motion sickness to the point of vomiting.

If the other symptoms were concerning and inconvenient, the vertigo, last to develop, was debilitating. Though its duration was usually no more than three to five minutes, he felt off for the rest of the day, like he was drifting through those eerie skies that follow a summer storm in the Midwest.

Convinced there was a diagnosis to explain this onslaught of vestibular distress, he was motivated to see providers and get help. He was proactive, starting with his PCP, then diligently scheduling specialist appointments with ear, nose, and throat doctors and allergists.

They sent him for CT scans, allergy shots, acupuncture, and chiropractic appointments. They sent scopes through his nostrils and ear canals to peer into the strange little apparatus that controls hearing and balance, something like a miniature amusement-park ride made up of delicate bones suspended above a tide pool. Apparently the root of Gabe's problems was that his "tide" was too high — excess fluid in his apparatus was causing pressure. Doctors advised a low-sodium diet, suggested plastic surgery to alter the roofs of his collapsed sinuses, and told him to avoid common allergens. All their advice was speculative and came with the caveat that these things may or may not help, may or may not be related.

So Gabe changed his lifestyle with commitment. He avoided dogs and pollen, swapped salted butter for its gloomy cousin. He followed up with integrated medicine, all the while remaining good-natured. He retained a level of optimism throughout that dizzy winter that impressed us all — because he was metaphorically running into walls, opening Murphy doors that led to nothing.

Little made a difference, and the bouts of vertigo started to come in closer succession. Pretty convinced he had Ménière's disease, a chronic condition with poorly understood etiology, he turned to the Internet for information he wasn't getting from the medical establishment. He wound up on message boards, reading threads that catastrophized the reality of Ménière's. He went down a hole and came back horrified.

It's difficult to reconcile Gabe's apparent vitality with chronic illness and debilitating pain. Following the Internet spiral, he wore trepidation on his person. "I never know when I'm going to have an attack," he explained, "but when I do I feel safer in my house, near my bed, where I can ride it out. I worry it will happen when I'm working. Actually, I always worry now. I'm hypersensitive and anticipate every little thing that could set it off and should therefore be avoided." It reflects the fears of many of my patients with chronic illness. The half-life of anticipation can be longer than the half-life of discomfort.

One day, a family member who worked nearby told him about a woman named Ellen who also had Ménière's. Gabe called her to set up a time to talk, which resulted in an hour-long phone call. Ellen was a stranger who became a vital source of reassurance and information on the realities of Ménière's: what not to worry about, the semihelpful to game-changing interventions, the medications to take and to avoid. She'd lived out some of his greatest worries about the disease. She became proof that a fulfilling life with Ménière's was not off the table.

Ellen was certainly a portal to hope when Gabe started to become hopeless, and she had advice and perspectives to offer that in many ways surpassed those of professional help.

While the idea of peer support runs counter to the way medical information was handled in earlier generations, when disease was not the stuff of dinner-table conversation but a private affair between patient and provider, our new impulse toward connecting has brought many new, sophisticated peer-support resources. These can link patients, even across large distances, in efforts to improve the course and outcome of chronic illnesses. Here are a few ways to access these resources:

Start with Your Providers

Just as you can ask doctors and nurses for patient references, you can ask if they know any patients with your condition who might be willing to talk with you. Providers and patients alike are generally willing to put forth effort to connect people under these circumstances. It fosters community.

Connect via the Internet

You can also use digital resources to access a variety of accounts of firsthand experiences with the disease or symptoms you're facing.

I advise against places like Reddit, since its threads weave a tangled web of contradictory information and malice that wavers on the edge of one big misery-loves-company party. The information isn't monitored, and one person's platform to vent shouldn't be another's source of data.

Instead, try http://www.patientslikeme .com. This site has a directory that works similarly to Facebook's, and you can use it to seek out people around the country who share your condition. The directory is set up to help patients interface both in public messaging forums and on a one-on-one basis. You can view individual profiles and create your own, with features like charts that highlight trends in your symptoms at various points along your disease trajectory.

You can also attend support groups in person. They're usually set up by patients, so they're free of ties to any professional or commercial interest. They're a good place for unbiased and helpful views on treatment options. The Office of Disease Prevention and Health Promotion has a search tool to find support groups in your area (https://healthfinder.gov/FindServices/SearchContext.aspx?topic=833).

ECONOMY OF DISEASE

In the event that you have a diagnosis, but the disease is less culturally recognized or understood, remember that you may need to be more intentional in asking for support.

In her piece "Cancer Is a Magic Word" in *Nightingale* magazine, writer Erica Schecter writes:

Having lived with ulcerative colitis for a decade, I thought I knew what it meant to be sick in the U.S. — but when I got cancer, I realized there's a hierarchy of disease. . . .

Say "I have cancer," and no one asks for explanations or justifications. Instead, they want to know all about the treatment side effects. I could miss as much work as I needed to. Friends flew out to visit me, left work to take me to chemo, and bought me books and games to make the long hours in the infusion suite pass more quickly. I was inundated with texts and calls, everyone just saying: "I'm here for you. Tell me what you need."

Earlier in the story, Schecter recounts the experience of receiving and living with a diagnosis of ulcerative colitis a decade prior. The inflammatory GI disease about which her friends and coworkers knew little and didn't have a framework for, in ways, had a more severe impact on her life than the cancer. This was in part because the disease didn't carry the same medical clout or instant recognition cancer carries with it.

Her story is a good reminder that it might take very intentional communication with friends, family, and peers if you suffer from a less well-known disease that takes a significant toll on your life. Remind yourself that they don't have an accessible framework to understand its impact and help you unless you reach out for support and explain. Solicit help with this from your nurses and providers, who can give you resources to assist in educating the people in your life about the condition, and give you ideas for how they can support you.

■ ■ ■ ■

Part V
When It's an
Emergency

■ ■ ■ ■

The following sections will ground you in emergency culture, so that you're equipped with a better decision-making tree when accidents happen. These are the "street emergencies" we're generally aware of and might recognize from television or have learned about in CPR training for babysitting. But beyond our general ability to recognize them, most of us feel helpless and paralyzed if they manifest. I hope this information primes you with a little muscle memory, so that if you witness a medical emergency you feel empowered to step in.

While these sections are not exhaustive, they include some of the most common medical emergencies you might encounter.

FOURTEEN:
ER VS. URGENT CARE VS. WAIT UNTIL MONDAY

Working in the medical profession comes with an unspoken agreement to answer calls and field texts from friends with medical questions. Nothing fazes me at this point. I've had lengthy discussions about vaginosis before I've finished my first coffee; woken up to texts with photos of rashes, abscesses, or ingrown hair follicles with strings of crying emojis; and been asked several times if X, Y, or Z warrants a trip to the ER. Even as a nurse I am not immune to this conundrum of what does and doesn't constitute an emergency. One summer, furiously deadheading an ancient English rosebush, I whacked my hand on the trunk and a thorn the size of a child's thumb went through and bashed one of the slender bones in the back of my hand. Thinking it might be fractured — and, since I was in the midst of taking clinical microbiology, sure I had contracted *Sporothrix schenckii,* rose gardener's disease — I indeed went to the ER because it was a Saturday afternoon. And I still want to kick myself for it.

At this fork in the road, with signs pointing to the emergency department, an urgent care center, or a U-turn back home to bed, most patients are at a loss, without resources to help them make a decision. Their best bet? The Internet. Phone a friend. Err on the side of caution.

These moments, when you're feeling like a shell of a human being, can cost either a lot of money to address, or a lot of suffering to wait out. And waiting it out can be dangerous: Without the appropriate antibiotic, an infection can linger indefinitely, especially in harsh winter conditions and when people are under stress. Wounds dealt with at home that actually required medical attention can become infected, putting people at risk for systemic problems. Fractures that go undiagnosed can heal improperly. Serious dehydration or an immune reaction sometimes just needs medical intervention.

On the other hand, it's likely that at one point or another you've regretted making the decision to go to the ER. You might have spent hours camped out in its various waiting rooms, finally advanced to a private exam room, and then waited endlessly for Dr. Schmoop to come in and tell you to take a high dose of ibuprofen, wasting you a good deal of time. Oh, and money! Emergency rooms are monopolies, and they take advantage of their market share. Take a hospital bill for services rendered and multiply it substantially, and you'll have an idea of what an average trip to the ER costs. For stitches, $1,200. For an MD to pat you on the head and send you on your merry way — or, in more generous terms, for peace of mind — $500 to $1,700.

There are times when an ER is absolutely necessary (we will identify many of them soon). There are also countless circumstances in which an urgent care facility is a better bet — less expensive, with shorter wait times.

THE DRAW OF THE ER

One of the first emergency departments in the United States was a two-bed facility at Johns Hopkins called the Accident Room. Patients were brought in via the town police wagon and treated free of charge. It all sounds idyllic compared to the chaotic holding pens we're familiar with today.

The function of emergency rooms today is a hot-button topic in the medical community, where industry leaders have made serious efforts to stem unnecessary visits. Insurance companies have gone so far as to refuse reimbursement when they deem an ER visit unnecessary. "Save the ER for emergencies — or cover the cost," reads a letter sent in 2017 to Blue Cross and Blue Shield customers of Georgia. "Going to the emergency room (ER) or calling 9–1–1 is always the way to go when it's an emergency. And we've got you covered for those situations." It continues, "But starting July 1, 2017, you'll be responsible for ER costs when it's not an emergency."[1]

The trend isn't a new one. For years US insurance companies have gotten away with denying claims based on the ultimate diagnosis when a patient goes to the ER. It means that if you have chest pain, think you're having a heart attack, go to an ER, and find out it's something nonurgent like a respiratory infection — you will be settled with the bill. First and foremost, this is unlawful, as the Prudent Layperson Standard, codified in federal law with the advent of the Affordable Care Act, states that reimbursement must be based on symptoms a patient is experiencing when they go to the ER, not the diagnoses. According to the American College of Emergency Physicians, insurance companies are taking advantage of political turmoil around the Affordable Care Act to push the envelope with these practices once again. It angers healthcare providers, this message sent on full blast to American patients that they're not to cry wolf or there will be consequences. It means someone might endure a stroke or a pulmonary embolism without going to an ER out of financial fears. To assume that the average patient can distinguish emergency from nonemergency situations confidently is unconscionable, as often even medical experts don't have this answer right away.

It's true that patients without established care often use the ER for nonemergencies, burdening the system and causing longer wait times for true medical emergencies. Industry leaders have made serious efforts to stem unnecessary visits for this reason.

For all its shortcomings when it comes to nonemergencies, the ER represents what is, to patients, the most direct path to care. It's a sensible point of access to the medical system for those who navigate it infrequently. Just as those who don't speak fluent French recognize the phrase "merci," patients who don't know whom to call or where to turn if they run a high fever still recognize an ER as a building that houses people and resources to help. The ER is a universal symbol. The luminescent red cross stands for "help."

It's interesting to look at the sources of information we call on to interpret the severity of a medical situation. Pain. Whatever medical knowledge we have. Memories of our past experiences, or the story of another's. Something we heard on the news or through the grapevine. It's frequently a combination of all the information traveling through our emotional brain and memory stores as we decide what to do and where to turn.

A better method starts with classifying emergent medical situations into three categories: **medical crises**, **emergencies**, and **urgent medical situations**. Doing so will help you get what you need efficiently and economically when you are in distress and need medical intervention. I've based the following sections on the triage system used in emergency departments.

CHOOSE THE ER IF . . .

Medical Crises

These are moments when individuals find themselves pinned between life and death. When your limb is lying next to you on the floor, or your lips are turning gray-blue, or your heart stops working. These include anything impacting the ABCs: airway, breathing, or circulation (see page 316). In situations like these, there's little decision-making to be done — call 911 and get to the nearest ER.

Emergencies

These fall slightly below medical crises. Not all are immediately fatal in nature but require equipment, procedures, or expertise only available in a hospital setting, and therefore warrant an emergency room visit. They're also typically time-sensitive. Examples include severe abdominal pain (which might indicate appendicitis) or deep lacerations. Remember that ER providers have a focused scope of practice relating to trauma and emergency, so ERs are typically not the place to seek a diagnosis for a chronic illness. Any diagnosis given in this setting should be reassessed by a specialist or discussed with your PCP.

Specific Situations

The following situations should send you to the emergency room immediately or to call 911:

Breathing that is compromised or difficult

Chest pain that is severe, radiating, of sudden onset, or accompanied by perspiration, shortness of breath, or nausea

Severe abdominal pain (of a nature markedly different from cramps or the average stomachache)

Severe pain in the lower back that intensifies with moderate finger pressure at the very bottom of the back

Sudden changes in mental status, balance, speech, or perception of language

Sudden paralysis, numbness, or weakness of a substantial portion of the body

An alteration in mental status that indicates the patient is at risk for harming themselves or others

Severe heart palpitations

Rapid swelling of any body part

Falls (in frail and/or elderly patients, especially if they take blood-thinning medications)

Sudden change in vision or loss of vision

Broken bone

Dislocated joint

Laceration that does not stop bleeding

after five to ten minutes while putting pressure on it

Head or eye injury

Severe burns

Seizure (when the patient does not have a history of seizures)

Severe flu with dehydration (see page 310)

Fever that climbs above 103° (for adults), lasts for more than two days with minimal response to OTC medications, or is accompanied by a rash

Fever of 100° or higher for a newborn baby

Vaginal bleeding during or after pregnancy

Unrelenting vomiting and diarrhea

The rule of thumb is that if what you're experiencing has a **sudden onset**, poses a threat to **basic functions** (ABCs or psychological functions), may lead to **losing a limb,** or is a physiological function that **changes rapidly** in a way that is foreign to you, you should go to the ER.

CHOOSE URGENT CARE IF . . .

Urgent Medical Situations

Urgent medical situations are those that cause you severe distress that won't subside without timely intervention. Ideally they would be addressed by a primary care provider or a specialist you see regularly, but when those resources aren't available quickly enough, you should go to urgent care. In a medical crisis *always* call 911, but if you're in doubt about a course of action for anything other than a medical crisis, look into an urgent care center.

Sometimes circumstances will leave you little choice between urgent care centers, but often you will have some flexibility in where you go. (See page 304 for how to choose the best ER for your situation.) Like ERs, urgent care centers vary in quality. Some are excellent, employing retired ER docs with loads of experience, while others are just set up to capitalize on low-lying fruits like colds. These aren't places to get a refined assessment or manage an acute manifestation of a complex illness. Before the need arises, locate a solid urgent care facility in your community (you can actually Yelp them to read reviews!) so you don't have to randomly pick one while holding a tourniquet to someone's arm. I went to an urgent care center with my friend just last summer and couldn't shake the feeling the place was a setup and everyone was playing hospital. There was something a bit Las Vegas about the whole joint — a flashy logo, a fancy front desk, bad art, and fake plants, but the exam rooms had cluttered cardboard boxes scattered around in corners and on the floor like a warehouse. And no sinks inside the exam room! The nurse in me died a small death.

Specific Situations

Situations that can be handled by urgent care include symptoms with a more gradual onset, symptoms causing you severe discomfort that cannot wait several days for aid, or minor injuries that can't wait for intervention:

Upper respiratory infection
Flu
Ear pain
Migraine
Pain or burning with urination
Persistent diarrhea
Swollen tonsils
Vomiting
Mild asthma

Broken bone of the wrist, hand, ankle, or
foot

Minor trauma, such as a common sprain
or shallow cut

CAN IT WAIT UNTIL MONDAY?

The decision here is ultimately personal,
but there are resources to help you make it.
The best way to determine if something can
wait is by contacting a medical professional.
If you have a primary care provider or care
established with a specialist — even if it's
been a while since you saw them — you
should call them and ask for advice if you're
not sure if you should go to the ER, urgent
care, or their office. If it's after-hours, they
may have a physician or nurse on call you
can speak to.

If you don't have an established PCP or
are unable to get through to or get advice
from your routine provider, try calling a
friend or relative in the medical field, if you
have one, and ask for their advice.

Many insurance plans include a free
telephone advice line staffed by nurses 24/7,
all trained to walk you through decisions
around medical emergencies. Some, like
Blue Cross, offer online doctor visits with a
$10 co-pay. They're available 24/7 and they
can offer prescriptions. This can be a help-

ful benefit to take advantage of if you're in a bind, can't get to a PCP, and want to avoid an urgent care trip.

A point that factors in here is that while something might be able to wait until the weekday for attention, your level of discomfort or your schedule may not allow that. If you don't have a PCP, finding one and setting up an intake appointment, then getting the issue addressed is unlikely to have a quick turnaround. Your PCP may not have availability. You may not be able to get to your clinic the coming weekdays as easily as you could on the weekend. As long as your situation does not fall within the medical crisis, emergency, or urgent medical situation parameters outlined above, factor these in as you make your decision, with or without the help of medical professionals via telephone.

EMERGENCY ROOM TIPS

Emergency Departments

The emergency department (ED) is the gatekeeper of the hospital, and most pathways to admission commence in its lobby. Beyond scheduled surgeries, only rare exceptions allow you to go around the ED. It's possible if you have a primary care provider advocating on your behalf and a condition that warrants urgent hospitalization for monitoring or stabilizing. In most cases, though, if you try to enter a hospital any other way you will be told flatly to go check yourself into the emergency department.

There, an ED doctor will review your case, run necessary scans and labs, and consult with a hospitalist or specialist to make a decision about whether you'll be admitted. Ensure that your primary care provider, the one who knows your health history, is looped into that conversation. If possible, call your provider's office en route to the hospital and ask them to call the ED prior to your arrival.

Choosing Your Emergency Room

In many emergency situations (such as broken bones or blunt traumas), your capacity to make decisions about where you're taken and who's consulted will be compromised. But in situations between minor and life-threatening, you may have the chance for some decision-making. When this is the case, take note of the following:

Every primary care provider has "privileges" at select hospitals. Gather this information about your PCP before there's an emergency. When there is an urgent situation, try to choose a hospital ED where, once you're admitted, your PCP will be able to see you and help manage your case.

It is extremely difficult to go through one hospital's ED and then get admitted to a different hospital. Choose an ED attached to a hospital you feel comfortable being admitted to, based on its trauma level, certifications, and proximity to your home.

For those with children: Designated pediatric EDs are much better equipped and trained to work with little ones — the cuffs and masks are miniature and the providers specialize in pediatrics. You can locate one at http://www.childrens hospitals.org.

In the Ambulance

This may come as a surprise, but you actually have a choice about which hospital an ambulance takes you to. When responders arrive, they will immediately assess you and determine if your condition is time-sensitive and/or life-threatening. If you're not incapacitated, you can request to be taken to a specific hospital, even if it's farther away. It may be worth slightly delaying treatment in order to go to a better hospital, or one where staff are familiar with your case. Exercising this option only makes sense if you're familiar enough with your condition and the ins and outs of the hospital systems in your community to make an informed decision. This might apply to cancer patients, elderly patients with chronic conditions, or patients with a condition that has exacerbations meriting a trip to a specific ED.

The paramedics will not be able to take you to a hospital that falls outside of their registered zone, or a hospital ER that is on divert and not taking new patients. If these are not obstacles and you still truly disagree with the paramedics' plan, you can ask to sign a waiver that relinquishes liability for the delay in treatment if you choose a hospital farther away. The message here: Paramedics are trained to strategize and get you to the place that can best attend to your emergency as quickly as possible. You can be involved in making this decision with them, but only in certain circumstances. It shouldn't come at the expense of distraction from the patient, or lost time.

FIFTEEN:
AM I DYING? (EMERGENCY PREPAREDNESS, EXTENDED)

GO TO THE ER, *RIGHT NOW!*

There are emergent situations that bring patients into the ER — chest pain, difficulty breathing, shooting abdominal pain — but there are also slow builds that warrant concern. Below are a host of situations — some medication-related and others related to allergens, hydration, and blood sugar — that should send you for immediate care.

ADVERSE MEDICATION REACTIONS

Advice from providers, pharmacists, drug labels, and drug commercials always seems to end with the same line: "Seek medical attention immediately if . . ." — followed by a host of random symptoms you're unlikely to remember. It's easy to become desensitized to the message, especially if you take several different medications with overlapping warnings. But a few situations really do warrant medical attention when you're on a new medication.

Situation One
A rash of red or purple spots that resemble blisters, and skin peeling on the body or blisters inside the mouth (with or without a fever)

Stevens-Johnson syndrome is an unpredictable reaction to medication (usually over-the-counter painkillers or antibiotics) that can cause sudden, massive skin sloughing that requires treatment in a burn unit if not addressed immediately. If you experience these symptoms, call your provider ASAP or head to the emergency room. If you've ever had this reaction, it's essential your medical providers know about it. Note that this one is quite rare, but serious and underestimated, so everyone should be aware of it.

Situation Two
Sudden itching in throat, and
Swelling tongue, and
Shortness of breath

These are classic signs of anaphylaxis (an extreme allergic reaction). It can happen without warning if your immune system rejects a medication or other environmental allergen. This requires immediate medical intervention — call the paramedics.

Situation Three
Change in mental status to agitation or confusion, and/or
Twitching or rigid muscles, and/or
Intense sweating, and/or
Dilated pupils

These changes are classic signs of an antidepressant gone awry. Serotonin syndrome can occur as the body adjusts to a new psychiatric medication, changes from one SSRI (selective serotonin reuptake inhibitor, a common type of antidepressant) to another, or tapers off an antidepressant. Call your doctor or go to an ER for assistance if one or more of these symptoms arises.

Situation Four
Not enough sugar.

Shakiness, damp skin, heart palpitations, and
Disorientation (the sensation of being drunk), and
Intense hunger

These are the classic signs of hypoglycemia (low blood sugar), which can be life-threatening to diabetics when severe. It's caused by too much insulin and not enough food to counter it. Immediately call for medical help and eat or drink juice, milk, or something sugary while you wait for them to arrive. This warrants an ambulance and paramedics.

Situation Five

Not enough water.

Use the following method to check for severe dehydration — whether the cause is food poisoning, a virus, or extreme heat.

Skin Tent:

Using the thumb and forefinger, pull up a small section of skin on the back of the hand. Under normal conditions, the skin will have elasticity and immediately slide back into place. If instead the skin stays up, forming a tent and then slowly slinking back down, the patient is severely dehydrated. Note that this test does not work with older adults, who have less elasticity to their skin.

If a positive skin tent test is paired with all the symptoms in the following list, it is time to go to the ER for fluid replacement:

Dry mouth

Sunken eyes (especially in children)
Dizziness or fainting
Low or halted urine output

If less severe signs of dehydration are present and you're able to drink fluids, you should drink broth, juice, or an electrolyte/sports drink. Do not drink solely water, unless it's the only thing available. Monitor your symptoms closely, and if they get worse or do not resolve with fluid intake, head in to the ER to be seen by a professional.

CARDIAC EMERGENCIES

Your heart will beat approximately 2.6 billion times in eighty years. It works hard. Heart disease causes more fatalities than any other medical condition — nationally, globally, and across sexes. Because of this, everyone should face it square on, understand how it operates, and be empowered with a plan if it happens to you or someone in your presence. Chances are, at some point in your life, it will.

While a heart attack can be an instantaneous, random, and circumstantial killer, it doesn't always come out of the blue. Concrete warning signs set the scene, so being aware and realistic about your risk of heart attack can enable you to save your own life.

311

First, you need to know where you fall on the risk continuum. The National Heart, Lung, and Blood Institute has outlined the following factors for increased risk. If three or more of these risk factors apply to you, you should create an action plan this week.

Risk Factors for Everyone

High blood pressure
High cholesterol
Diabetes or prediabetes
Smoking
Being overweight or obese
Being physically inactive
Family history of heart disease
Unhealthy diet
Age, being 65 or older

Risk Factors Specific to Women

History of preeclampsia during pregnancy
Endometriosis
Being postmenopausal
Having polycystic ovarian syndrome

See page 473 for a full discussion on sex differences in heart attack presentation and treatment.

Prevention and First Aid

If you have three or more risk factors, regardless of your sex, you should be tested for ischemia (the heart attack's cousin that often shows up first) and coronary artery disease (CAD). Ischemia can be silent and asymptomatic, but if it's tested for and accurately diagnosed, you can set a plan in motion that gives you the best chance at preventing or surviving a heart attack. This is especially important for women.

Sublingual nitroglycerin and aspirin can both help in the event of a suspected heart attack. Ask your provider if you should keep a dose on hand and how to use. Based on your medical profile you'll likely benefit more from one than the other, but each of these medications can relax the blood vessels, giving you some time to get to a professional.

You should also have a paper list of all medications, vitamins, and supplements you take (see page 125) and — this one is important and overlooked — a copy of your resting EKG. Hand these to the emergency team, or assign the responsibility to a family member or your advocate, if you present somewhere with what you believe to be a heart attack.

Who to Tell

The people around whom you spend the most time should know a) that you carry risk and b) that they should *not* attempt to drive you anywhere, but rather should call 911 if you suddenly exhibit signs of extreme physical distress. This is critical, because pulling up to the ER in a private vehicle does not get you the same swift delivery of care as arriving in an ambulance. When you take an ambulance, your treatment also begins en route to the hospital.

In Case of a Suspected Heart Attack

Who to Call
Your plan of action in the event of a suspected heart attack is as follows: Call 911, say you believe you're having a heart attack, and wait. Even if the symptom isn't traditionally associated with heart attacks or you feel okay otherwise, don't attempt to drive yourself to the hospital. Don't call your regular provider or clinic before calling 911.

Once You're at the ER
Ensure you're given an EKG and a troponin test, which looks for tiny bits of damaged heart muscle in your blood. If both are normal but you don't have a satisfying

diagnosis that explains your symptoms — and especially if they have not resolved — get a second opinion from a cardiologist ASAP.

SIXTEEN:
ARE THEY DYING?
(PEDESTRIAN EMERGENCIES)

Nobody text me in a crisis.

— RIHANNA

IN THESE SITUATIONS,
TIME IS OF THE ESSENCE

If you think you are witnessing any of the following situations, time is extraordinarily important, so never wait before calling 911:

Stroke
Heart attack
Anaphylaxis
Severe blood loss
Persisting asthma attack

If in doubt, think about the ABCs. If any one of them is in jeopardy, call 911 immediately:

Airway: If the airway is blocked by swelling or a foreign object

Breathing: If the person is not taking between twelve and twenty breaths per minute

Circulation: If, due to blood loss or an obstruction the naked eye can't see, blood is not getting to the organs — this is hard to determine out in the world, but can be indicated by pain or a change in pallor, like the skin turning blue

IF YOU WITNESS AN EMERGENCY

Disco CPR

If you are presented with the opportunity to save a life, we'll assume you'll take it — or at least give it a college try. But when we see someone lose their pulse, many of us will freeze in the ensuing chaos and fear. Here are tips to help better prepare you.

First, ask the nearest person to call 911. If it's only you and the downed person, call before you do anything else.

Next, take the advice of the American Heart Association and look to the Bee Gees for help: Place the base of your palm on the nipple line. Then place your hands one on top of the other, with interlocked fingers. Focusing weight on the base of your palm, start hands-on compressions over the chest cavity to the beat of "Stayin' Alive." Truly! Everyone knows the beat of this song, and it's the exact tempo needed to deliver the recommended one hundred beats per minute.

Rescue breaths should always come secondary to compressions. When you're giving those compressions, you're also causing the lungs to contract and expand, so if you're the only one on the scene, always prioritize compressions. If you choose to give rescue breaths in addition, give two breaths after every thirty chest compressions: Tilt the person's head back, plug their nose, cover their mouth with yours entirely like you're blowing up a balloon, and give two breaths. Then, immediately go back to compressions. If another person is present, you can share these roles and switch off. If the individual is a stranger, you're *not* expected to give mouth to mouth CPR without protective equipment.

Real-life CPR (cardiopulmonary resuscitation) is nothing like the movies. If you know this, you're already a step ahead. People don't always realize that in order for this intervention to work, all those chest compressions need to literally reach the heart. If you've never done it, the force you'll need to use is probably more intense than you'd think. Sometimes it will cause fractures. I bring this up not to scare you but to reiterate the force needed to get the blood circulating. CPR can sometimes be ineffective because it's too gentle!

When done properly, CPR will wear you out. It can be very physically exhausting, so call out for help if anyone is around, tell them what to do, and switch off with them. Just remember:

30 compressions
2 breaths
Saturday Night Fever

Quick Tips if You Witness a Seizure

With seizures, the thing that feels intuitive to do might actually run counter to what should be done to help. If the person hasn't had a seizure before (or if you don't know), or if the person is or appears pregnant, first call 911. Your next steps:

If the person is standing, gently lower them to the floor.

Clear the surroundings of furniture or other obstructive objects.

Roll the person on their side to prevent

319

aspiration (choking).

Don't try to hold the person down to protect them. This can cause injury.

Do not put anything in the person's mouth.

Time the seizure if you can. (This might seem odd, but it's very helpful for medical professionals to know the duration.)

Keep the person calm and safe, staying with them for at least thirty minutes post-seizure.

Quick Tips if You Witness a Severe Allergic Reaction

Anaphylaxis is the mother of all allergic reactions. It can come on like lightning and, if not treated, can be fatal within thirty minutes. Typically when we think of an allergic reaction, we think of hives, redness, and itching. Anaphylaxis, however, is characterized by these things plus a cascade of swelling, difficulty breathing, and sometimes nausea and vomiting. But mostly swelling which, as it progresses in the throat and airways, cuts off breathing.

Other signs of anaphylaxis include:

Wheezing
Itching, burning, or tingling skin
Rapid heartbeat
Loss of consciousness

In these situations, the patient needs an EpiPen immediately. When in doubt, always administer an EpiPen. Better safe than sorry in cases of anaphylaxis — it's much worse not to give it when it's needed than to give it when it's not warranted. If there's no EpiPen on hand, though, call 911 immediately. Be sure to tell the operator that you believe the person you're with is experiencing anaphylaxis. The time frame for treating anaphylaxis before things get very dicey is thirty minutes, so don't delay seeking emergency help.

If you do use an EpiPen, keep in mind:

Know how to use it *before* an emergency strikes. Read the instructions and get comfortable with the procedure. (It's injected into the outer thigh.)

Always check the expiration date. Set a reminder on your calendar to replace the pen before its expiration date.

Stay alert for recalls. Set an alert on Google News so you'll get an email any time an EpiPen recall pops up.

The generic option is less expensive and can save you upward of $300 for two pens. Ask your pharmacist about it.

Quick Tips if You Witness a Stroke

There are multiple schools of thought on how to recognize a stroke as it's happening, but I think the best out there — and the easiest to remember — is the FAST acronym from the National Stroke Association. It's the one I share with my own patients and family.

Remember the Word FAST

Face: Ask the person to smile. Does one side of the face droop?

Arms: Ask the person to raise both arms. Does one arm drift downward?

Speech: Ask the person to repeat a simple sentence. Are the words slurred? Can he/she repeat the sentence correctly?

Time: If the person shows any of these symptoms, time to call 911.

Other Symptoms Include Sudden:

Numbness or weakness of the face, arm, or leg, especially on one side of the body

Confusion, trouble speaking or understanding

Trouble seeing in one or both eyes

Trouble walking, dizziness, loss of balance or coordination

Severe headache with no known cause

Unique Symptoms of Strokes in Women Can Include:

A sudden and out-of-character change in mental status

Nausea and vomiting

Seizures

Hiccups

Difficulty breathing

Sudden pain or weakness

Fainting

Whether the above occur in tandem or show up on their own without a sound explanation, call for help. The acronym is FAST for a reason, so be quick. Time is especially of the essence when brain tissue is at stake.

PART VI
WHEN YOU'RE
HAVING A
PROCEDURE

■ ■ ■ ■

Much like how the blood rushes to your stomach after you eat, once you're recommended to have a procedure all attention and concern can divert to getting through it. This means patients might end up leaving to chance decisions that are better addressed at the outset.

Doing some work on the front end is worth it — to ensure that a procedure is necessary, it's performed by a skilled person, and you understand in plain language what will go down in the operating room and the possible outcomes. Just as important, you should try to make sure that variables like the day, time, and place your provider sets for the procedure do not cause you to incur a significantly larger bill.

The following section will guide you through simple practices that will streamline medical interventions and ensure that they are as safe, effective, and economic as possible.

SEVENTEEN:
CHOOSING IF, WHERE, AND WHO

SECOND OPINIONS

According to the multiverse theory, there is an infinite number of other universes that coexist with the one before us. Meaning there's a version of you who never left Kansas. One who dropped everything for the adventure, or didn't. A version who held onto your dream of becoming an oil painter and is now in overalls on a porch in Taos. A version who arrived at the bar ten minutes later and never met that person who altered your life in some profound way.

The multiverse theory is also at play when we're patients. Though we like to think medicine is an exact science, it's subjective, and second opinions are an incredible testament to this fact. It's estimated that upward of 60 percent of second opinions result in a different diagnosis or course of treatment — yet many patients don't pursue them. This makes medicine look more like a serendipitous chain reaction than an exact science — the decisions tenuous, the outcomes dependent on instinct, time, and place.

Upwards of one fifth of all surgeries performed in the United States are unnecessary, as are one third of elective surgeries (those that are scheduled in advance, instead of done during an emergency).[1] It's easy to glaze over the numbers, but consider that if you and three of your family members have surgery in the coming years, one of those surgeries will likely have been unnecessary. There's also a one-in-three chance that a colleague of the surgeon who operates would have taken another course of action. That's how often medical professionals disagree on complex matters.

Even with second opinions, there will be risks to calculate, and decisions that come down to gut and instinct. Still, I recommend getting the additional opinions. Take the chance to glimpse the multiverse and see a few possible outcomes before embarking.

Don't Worry About Offending Your Provider

Second opinions are a standard of practice, a matter of routine for all medical professionals. Many patients think that asking for another opinion will directly challenge the person they've already placed trust in, and many worry it will result in a compromised relationship and subpar treatment should they decide to stick with the original plan. Shed this complex! Medical professionals certainly seek out other opinions for themselves and their loved ones, so this concern for their ego is unfounded. Your health and safety come first, and humility should be a trait in any medical professional you're trusting with your body.

Timing Matters

Some patients avoid getting a second opinion out of anxiety about time. When you find out something is wrong, you may want it out, eradicated, addressed as soon as possible. It makes sense. Still, stop and get another set of eyes on your situation. Don't let time dissuade you from taking this route.

Who to See

A general rule of thumb when looking for another opinion is to avoid bias. This means not taking a recommendation from your first provider (though some might disagree here). Many hospitals now offer second opinions online, but whether they're a formality designed to make money or adequately thorough depends on the quality of the program and institution.

I advise taking the matter into your own hands. Do some research and find another specialist, ideally one in another hospital network. You can ask friends in the industry or employees at other hospitals (see page 340 for how to find the right surgeon), and use the online tools referenced in this book.

What Will It Cost?

Many insurance plans cover second opinions. If you are, in fact, one of those 34 percent of people who do not need a procedure, it's much less expensive for the insurance company to cover the cost of a second opinion than that of the procedure. It's in everyone's best interest. If the second opinion is deemed medically necessary, most insurance plans will pay at least part of the cost. Medicare will pay 80 percent of the cost and, if the second opinion doesn't agree with the first, 80 percent of the cost of a third opinion.[2]

Some plans have more comprehensive coverage than others, and for some you will need a referral from your PCP, so call and get the details of what your plan offers before you commence the search.

At the Appointment

Bring your medical records, with the most recent notes from your first assessment at the top of the pile. Do not assume the second provider has read up on the case; ensure the information is readily accessible to them so they can review it in front of you.

You certainly don't need to sit in silence, but you also don't need to go into great detail about the first opinion, or attempt to dissuade the provider from going in a certain direction. Answer questions and communicate your priorities toward the end of the discussion, but give the provider space to view the case through the most objective lens possible.

Now What?

If the second opinion corroborates the diagnosis of your initial evaluation, you can proceed with a newfound sense of confidence. If the opinions conflict significantly, it's advisable to go for a third. It varies case by case, and you'll have to tap into your own intuition and the specifics of your situation here. At a certain point, continuing to get opinions will stall things too long and start to introduce noise that could dissuade you from taking the best course of action.

Use your best judgment.

Second Opinions Are Not Just for Procedures

This one tends to surprise patients, but surgeries and invasive treatment plans are not the only medical interventions for which you can get second opinions. Radiology interpretations (of CT scans, MRIs, and X-rays) are also vulnerable to errors and subjectivity — radiologists even frequently disagree with their own interpretation of slides when they assess them a second time. Any time you are given a major diagnosis based on one of these scans or tests and your team isn't 100 percent sure, you can ask that the slides are sent for another opinion, such as to a nationally recognized lab for a second or third evaluation. Contacting a professor of radiology at an academic institution near you might also help guide you in where to send the slides.

RECON

When you want to be convinced, beyond a reasonable doubt, that the procedure is the best option for you, you'll need to do some reconnaissance. Here's a mnemonic I came up with to remember questions you should always ask in conversations about surgeries and procedures:

R (risks and benefits): What are the risks and benefits?

E (experience): What is your experience/success rate with this procedure?

C (cost): What will it cost and why?

O (other options): What other options do I have?

N (nothing): What are the risks of doing nothing, compared to the risks of the procedure?

How to Choose a Hospital

We all value different things during a medical encounter, including a hospital stay. One person might hate the thought of being referred to in the third person while a herd of students crowds their room, while another person might love the attention and the opportunity to be part of the educational process. While a hospital's proximity to home or a support network might matter greatly for an elderly couple because one will be going home each night during the hospital stay, others might send this to the bottom of their list.

There's a good bit of nuance that comes with choosing where to have your procedure. First, know that *you* have the ultimate say in where you go. Use the tips below to help you make a sound decision on the best setting for your care.*

Quality

When it comes to the quality of care you'll receive at a given hospital, the issue is twofold: how successful the surgery will be, and how you will be cared for before, during, and after.

A simple rule of thumb is that the more times a procedure has occurred at that hospital, the more successful the procedure will be. You can look up these rates across all zip codes using CareChex (http://www.carechex.com), which factors in not only the hospital's quality for performing your particular procedure but also how it ranks overall in safety and quality.

Certain types of hospitals are also better for certain types of procedures. Say, for instance, you're having a tonsillectomy and want to go to the big, sparkling academic

* These same principles can be applied to outpatient clinics where procedures take place.

hospital on the hill because you want the best. It's possible your boring (to them) little procedure might get lost in the shuffle. Remember all the moaning on *ER* when the residents got assigned to the appendectomy instead of the Whipple? There's a reason! There's a lot of glamour to the cutting edge, the novel, at hospitals like those, and they might not be the best choice for something common if you want the most attentive team. This isn't a reason not to have a procedure there, but one that should prompt you to consider other options as well. Don't choose a hospital because of the research wings being erected across campus. Rather, look up the statistics about the procedure you're getting using an independent source like the one previously listed.

The second issue, how you will be treated after the procedure, is equally important. It's easy to think you're willing to compromise bedside service for a world-renowned surgeon or state-of-the-art technology, but these things do not always translate to better care if the hospital misses the mark on postoperative follow-up. (See "The Importance of Follow-Up Care," page 355, for a story.)

Type of Facility

Outpatient, ambulatory surgical clinics can be a good option if you want to avoid hospitals altogether and your procedure can take place outside of one. But it's important to discuss a backup plan with the doctors there in case there's a complication during the procedure, as most clinics don't have emergency facilities. Where is the closest emergency center or full-scale hospital? What is their step-by-step plan of getting you treatment if you have a stroke or heart attack while in their care, or if something else happens that's beyond their expertise? These are questions to ask.

Political

This country has both for-profit and not-for-profit hospitals, and while they handle tax write-offs differently, both are rolling in the dough. I recently visited a hospital whose lobby had glass floors with crystal-line streams and tiny fish running underneath, and collections of paintings adorning the walls that might as well have been on loan from the Louvre. The hospital also boasted an established chef running the "dietary program" (which means a chef designed some foolproof recipes that could be produced on a mass scale and styled for photos). And, like other hospitals of its kind, it was erected recently in an affluent, suburban setting — meaning because of the cruel reality of residential segregation in our country, it's inaccessible to people of lower socioeconomic status. It means those fountains and paintings were bought with a huge sum of tax dollars that could have gone to helping people in the community who couldn't afford an emergency visit or a checkup.

Politics alone shouldn't determine your decisions, nor would I judge anyone for receiving a procedure from a great surgeon at this hospital. But in the current social climate, many of us are reconsidering the ways small, seemingly benign decisions reinforce societal systems of oppression. It's fair to consider these issues, or at least be aware of them.

Price

Price is the determining factor for most of us. This book includes a simple five-step process you can use to determine what your procedure would cost at each location you're considering — and they could vary exponentially. Head to "Healthcare Bluebook," page 526, for more information.

One last thing: You don't have to make your final decision sight unseen. You can ask to tour a unit or outpatient clinic where the procedure will take place. Call and set it up beforehand, and you can get a feel for the facilities and staff before committing to a procedure there. Simply remember this is another aspect of your healthcare about which you have a say. Don't just let someone tell you where and when to show up!

CARE PATHWAYS

We can thank Sweden for IKEA, ABBA, H&M, and gravlax — and better surgical outcomes.

In 2010, the Enhanced Recovery After Surgery (ERAS) Society was established in Stockholm. Its goal was to improve care and avoid complications during commonly performed surgeries by reviewing research and designing more refined care pathways. Its first program was implemented at Örebro University Hospital to great success, and the initiative was brought overseas in early 2016.

These programs are already starting to show promise for their ability to shorten hospital stays and recovery times and reduce the incidence of complications in US hospitals. Today, an ERAS care pathway signifies that a hospital has redesigned their standard of care for a procedure based on a national, comprehensive review of the literature on outcomes in pain management, patient stress, length of stay, and common complications.

The protocol uses multidisciplinary input from surgeons, hospitalists, nurses, physical therapists, and social workers to develop a plan around a surgery. Think of it as a redistribution of weight along the care continuum of a procedure: The crescendo of attention is typically on the table, in the operating room, but this model gives equal consideration to preoperative, postoperative, and recovery periods. The bar is set as high for pain control, infection prevention, and return to quality of life as it is for successful surgery.

Let's take the example of a knee-replacement surgery. The day after such surgeries, patients typically experience intense and only moderately controlled pain. The hospital stay usually lasts three to four days. In contrast, the ERAS program uses a novel eleven-point pain scale designed specifically to manage postoperative knee pain. The new care pathway, composed of this knee pain scale and other customized interventions, has been shown to reduce pain drastically, with one in three patients reporting no pain throughout the entire hospital stay. The ERAS program also reduces the stay to fifteen hours. I don't think it's a stretch to say that these programs can have as much impact as the expertise of the surgeon.

Care pathways are gradually being adopted in American hospitals across various specialties, but it will take time before they're widely accessible. As you consider different locations for your procedure, you can call around and see what institutions in your area offer care pathway programs. The list is evolving rapidly.

HOW TO CHOOSE A SURGEON

If you're seeking a second opinion or moving forward with an elective procedure, you may have a sea of potential surgeon candidates. Here are some tools to help you find the best match.

First and foremost, check the Federation of State Medical Boards (http://www.fsmb.org) to ensure that any surgeon you're considering is licensed, without sanction.

Review the surgeon's complication and

success rates. The sites http://www
.surgeonratings.org and http://projects
.propublica.org/surgeons allow you to
access detailed information about surgeons in your zip code based on their
success rate with various common procedures.

Ask the staff at the hospital where they
practice for recommendations. Do you
have a friend or relative who works for
the institution and can ask for you or
connect you with someone on the floor?
Do you know any nurses who would be
willing to do some reconnaissance? If
not, you can cold-call the unit yourself,
explain your situation, and ask if they
recommend any particular surgeons.

Ask the surgeon if you can talk to their
former patients. While HIPAA (a
confidentiality-protection law) prevents
surgeons from giving out contact information, they might have a past patient
or two who would be amenable to speaking with you, and they could connect
you after confirming. This is a courtesy
on the provider's part, as it takes additional work, but it's a standard request

and any good surgeon is likely to grant it.

Once You've Chosen

Before any major surgery, schedule meetings to tour the unit where you will be cared for before and after the surgery, and to meet the surgeon in person. Enlist your primary care provider's help to request this appointment, or call the office yourself. State that you'd like fifteen minutes with the surgeon to go over things sometime in the week or days leading up to the surgery. Also try to meet with the anesthesiologist assigned to your care.

Questions for Your Surgeon

Briefly go over your medical history. Then ask:

Which complications are they most concerned about?

What is the plan to address postoperative pain or nausea?

Who will oversee your care in the hospital after surgery? Will they be accessible after surgery, and how will they be reachable? (For example, if your surgery is on a Thursday, are they working over the weekend? If they aren't available, who will be covering?

(If it's a teaching hospital) Will they be performing the surgery themselves, or standing by while a resident performs it?

Questions for Your Anesthesiologist
Ask for fifteen minutes with your anesthesiologist to:

Do a thorough review of your medical history.

Get assurance that they will be in the room with you for the duration of the procedure.

Ask how any special circumstances (e.g., if you're frail or have allergies to standard anesthesia formulas) will be addressed.

THE DAYS LEADING UP TO A PROCEDURE

The week leading up to a major procedure is one of strange weather. If you've been there, I imagine you can recall the time with particular clarity.

343

I tell my patients that this is a time to be gentle with yourself. It's a highly personal task — it can't be prescriptive — but it should involve things that help you feel settled and place a few coins of resilience in your back pocket for when they're needed.

If the surgery is scheduled (nonemergency), let your primary care provider know that you're having it. Doing so will create a channel for better communication between you and your primary care provider, as well as between your primary care provider and the surgeon. For example, since your PCP knows your history more thoroughly, they might advocate for taking you off of a medication prior to surgery. Two heads are better than one, and if your PCP has knowledge of the surgery they can add additional insight and support to the case. This communication will also pave the way for more coordinated follow-up care once you're released from the hospital.

It's also a time to connect with your advocate, and/or the other friends and family who will be around. On one of the days leading up to checking in (perhaps not the evening prior to your procedure, since that's typically colored by anxiety or Xanax), schedule a game-plan discussion with your person or people. (If you do not know who to turn to in this situation, see page 112 for tips and resources on identifying and appointing an advocate.)

Compile the following information about your procedure. Make copies available for each person who will be around, or send it via email.

Details

Place (including the unit you will be admitted to and returned to after surgery), date, time, and expected duration of the procedure

The procedure itself and the specific condition it is treating (e.g., lumpectomy for tubular carcinoma of the breast, Stage II)

People

The names of the surgeon, anesthesiologist, and any other specialists directly involved in the procedure

The name of the charge nurse who will be working on the unit to which you will be admitted after the procedure (you can call the unit to get this information a few days ahead of time)

Medications

A comprehensive list of the medications you take daily and that you should be taking while in the hospital

A list of medications commonly prescribed for use before and after your procedure, and what they're for (you can find this information online, or ask your provider's office for a list — you can also enter the condition on http://www.drugs.com/condition to see which drugs are commonly used to treat it)

Any serious to life-threatening side effects to be aware of for each medication (you can look them up at http://www.drugs.com/sfx)

Complications

This section rests on a discussion with your provider (which can be done as soon as the procedure is scheduled), plus some brief, supplemental Internet research. In this section, list out any complications associated with the procedure, and how to recognize their signs.

This sounds daunting, but all the information is there — you just need to compile and distill it. Then you can use it to have a conversation with your advocate, friends, and family. Here's an example that should illuminate the task and show you it's more simple than it sounds.

Details

I am having a coronary artery bypass surgery at Cedar Sinai Hospital, unit 5A, this coming Thursday. The surgery is scheduled for 7 a.m. and expected to last four hours.

The bypass surgery is an intervention for a plaque in my coronary artery that needs to be circumvented. The surgeon will go in and graft a vein around the blockage so blood can flow more easily.

People

Cardiothoracic surgeon: Martha Rush
Anesthesiologist: Kasra Shokat
Vascular surgeon: Tess Tumarkin
Charge nurse: Gabriel Zinn (unit direct line: 503-555-0142)
PCP: Jillian Porten (office number: 503-555-0101)

Medications

Daily, I take:
Vitamin D, 200 units
Lexapro, 50 mg
Lotensin, 40 mg
Inderal, 25 mg
Baby aspirin, 81 mg
New medications that might be used during this stay, and potential adverse side effects to keep an eye out for:
IV morphine (for pain): dizziness, slowed breathing, constipation
Phenergan (for nausea): dizziness, ringing in ears
Coumadin (to control bleeding): severe bleeding, blood in urine
Pepcid (to protect stomach lining): dizziness, weakness, constipation, or diarrhea

Complications
Clot forms after surgery, causing heart attack, stroke, or pulmonary embolism
Watch for: Irregular activity on heart monitor, chest pain, face drooping, arm weakness, speech slurring, sudden confusion, shortness of breath, chest pain

Internal bleeding

Watch for: Sharp stomach pain, shortness of breath, decreased blood pressure (so, watch my vitals)

Infection of chest wound

Watch for: Any signs of infection in the wound, fever, rapid pulse, unusually low body temperature, vomiting, diarrhea

If any of these happens: Alert my assigned nurse. Alert Gabriel Zinn, the charge nurse, and ask him to page surgeon Martha Stevenson, who is overseeing the case. If there is no response within thirty minutes, call the rapid response line and request an evaluation: 503-555-0001.

Once you've made the list, go over it with your advocate and see if they have any questions. This will prime them for any common complications they should be on the lookout for, and empower them to ask questions. It's not to make them (or you) nervous or anticipate disaster, but to instill a deeper sense of confidence, preventing a situation where everyone goes in blind and has to address problems reactively.

INFORMED CONSENT

Us: Blah blah blah.

You, as the patient, nod, and look like you're paying close attention.

Us: Did you understand everything we said?

You: Yes.

Us: Any questions?

You: No.

There's a sort of collusion that takes place, and we're all complicit.

— MIKKAEL A. SEKERES
AND TIMOTHY D. GILLIGAN,
NEW YORK TIMES

Informed consent is meant to inform patients of the risks and benefits of medical interventions. It serves this function, sometimes successfully and sometimes not so successfully, but it also protects surgeons, doctors, practitioners, and hospitals against malpractice.

Providers want you to understand the risks and benefits of a procedure — its potential alternatives, the likelihood it will have the intended outcome, the result of not going forth with the intervention, and the worst-case scenarios. To skip this step would be to rip the medical code of ethics asunder. Whether or not they communicate these in a way you can understand is another matter.

Signing an informed consent form indicates that you understand all aspects of the medical intervention, and you're making a voluntary choice to proceed with it. If the provider is rushed, if you are anxious, and if communication is tenuous, you may assume that — like with most medical forms — you're being *told* to sign this rather than asked. Informed consent cannot take place under these circumstances, however, regardless of whether or not you signed.

Informed consent is black-and-white: Do you have free will? Given the outlined information, do you give consent to proceed? You, as a patient, are responsible for covering the gray area in between. Under proper informed consent, you navigate that territory with the help of your provider.

If you are up for a big procedure, surgery, or medical intervention (such as chemotherapy), schedule the informed-consent discussion, when you will sign the sheet, a few days to a week before the procedure itself. This limits the effects of urgency and anxiety on your ability to make decisions. It also gives you time to look into alternative options, get a second opinion if you want to, or talk to another patient who has gone through the intervention. This is also a good time to look into the hospital's record and the surgeon's record around the procedure (see pages 334 and 342).

Your safety is more important than the provider's time. Do not feel rushed to sign, even if your questions are met with a look of impatience or skepticism — or even if you're scheduled to be in surgery within the hour.*

Only providers can discuss informed consent. Fight the urge to ask a nurse or therapist their opinion, as they are legally and ethically prohibited from providing it.

You never have to sign away your rights. You do have to sign the form in order to be admitted, but you can modify it as you like. Writing "I am forced to sign in order to get treatment for condition X, but I do not relinquish my rights willfully" can protect you later if malpractice occurs.

Ask any questions you have. Even if they seem outlandish, even if you've already discussed them last week in your doctor's office but want to go over them again. If

---

* This does *not* apply to emergency situations, or other situations where waiting is high risk and ill-advised.

you can't think of questions, explain back to the provider what you understand will happen. This is the same as the teach-back method and can be as simple as this:

"I understand that I have _____ and am moving forward with _____ because it's going to _____. I also understand that _____ could happen if I proceed, and _____ could happen if I don't."

Only once the above items have been covered should you move forward.

There's no such thing as an off-limits question when it comes to ethical informed consent. The medical community set up this system to empower patients, protect their dignity, and respect the decision-making process. It can only function if you're an active party in the process.

RIGHT BEFORE SURGERY

If you've had major surgery, it's likely you've been hit over the head with the rules. No food after midnight. Do not shave with a razor beforehand. (Anywhere! It leaves you prone to infection.) Stop those medications. Start these. Get an incredible, restorative night's sleep beforehand, and, oh yes, arrive at 5 a.m. for prep.

To balance it out, here are a few things *you* are going to ask from your care team to ensure not only that things go well on the operating table, but also that you're as comfortable as possible post-op.

The priority of any surgery — be it to remove an appendix or fix a leaking aortic valve — is a successful operation. After that, the most pressing concern on every patient's mind before entering an operating room is pain — what to anticipate, how to avoid it, how to control it. But pain tends to take up so much of the conversation that it's easy to sideline something that can be just as miserable — postoperative nausea and vomiting (PONV). Planning is key, as treating PONV preemptively is more effective than treating it at its onset. Approximately one in three of us might experience PONV after surgery, thanks to a combination of our physiological makeup, the anesthesia cocktail that's been coursing through us, and the painkillers that disturb the GI tract. Females, nonsmokers, those who get motion sickness, and those taking opioids are at increased risk for PONV.

If these apply to you, let your surgeon or anesthesiologist know. Also keep in mind that gynecological, abdominal, and inner-ear surgery are associated with some of the highest rates of PONV. To prevent PONV, your provider will apply a patch before the surgery and give you a regimen of antiemetics post-op.

If you're having major surgery and anticipate substantial pain, ask your provider if you're eligible for a PCA pump. This is a patient-controlled opioid pump (it stands for "patient-controlled analgesia") that allows you to control when and how much pain medication is dispensed. It's hooked up to the IV and a small control button rests in the bed. In cases of major surgery, it's important to stay on top of pain to the best extent possible, but often a patient's ability to communicate pain and a nurse's ability to manage it at every turn are compromised. While the option isn't suitable for everyone — such as patients with a history of opioid addiction, or complex cases with too many medications on board to allow flexibility with pain intervention — it's worth discussing with your surgeon.

THE IMPORTANCE OF FOLLOW-UP CARE

He was the best. He'd operated on Pavarotti! It was like being in the presence of a demigod. Sure, there were moments we questioned his judgment . . . but we never questioned *him.* When I look back . . . I

should have made something happen.
— AN INTERVIEW WITH PHYLLIS MOSSBERG,
MY MEEMA, NEW YORK, 2018

Ten years ago, Phyllis lost her husband, Sandy, to postoperative complications. A few months before the surgery, he was diagnosed with a rare type of cancer in the islet cells of his pancreas. While the prognosis for pancreatic cancer is typically grim, islet-cell tumors tend to be less aggressive, and patients often go into remission once the tumor is removed. A gastroenterologist himself, Sandy was optimistic, and so was his family.

He knew the success of the operation hung on finding an excellent surgeon, so he and his family searched until they found the best. Dr. A had a reputation that preceded him on the East Coast. As the family describes it, receiving him — with a swarm of residents on his tail — at NewYork-Presbyterian/Columbia University Medical Center (one of New York's best teaching hospitals) was nothing short of ceremonious.

"He's in recovery. It was a huge success. The tumor virtually popped out," he told the family while Sandy recovered in post-op.

Soon after, Sandy was moved to a rehabilitation unit on the basement floor of the hospital. Around this time things began to unravel as staff stopped communicating with one another.

The first incident happened a few mornings into his stay in the basement, when Phyllis was en route to the hospital and got a call from her husband. He told her he was having chest pain.

"It was hard to get people to come down to that floor," she recalls, especially the team who oversaw his surgery and knew his case. She finally got the attention of a fourth-year resident.

"He poked his head in," she recalls, "not his whole body but just his little head. And he said it was probably just a pulled muscle."

"I was pushy," she says. "I was not worried about being loved by anyone."

"Young man," she said, "this is a person in his seventies with chest pain and you're chalking it up to a pulled muscle? Let's come back in here. All the way."

Sandy did not have a pulled muscle — he had a collapsed lung and needed immediate intervention.

That same week, Meema stopped a nurse from mistakenly giving Sandy Coumadin, a blood thinner that would have caused him to bleed out in his condition. At another point, when Sandy was in physical therapy in a separate wing of the hospital, his vitals started to deteriorate and staff called a code blue — but no one came. It wasn't until twenty-four hours later that Sandy's surgical team arrived and finally intervened to bring his vitals back up. They defended their absence by explaining that the physical therapy unit was technically not part of the hospital, so they were unavailable to respond to the code in the same way.

Sandy and Phyllis' daughters, Amy and Julie, recall that the anticipated postoperative weakness went on for longer than anyone expected. It took great effort for Sandy to swallow, and he didn't have the strength to eat much of anything. This didn't seem to concern anyone — until Sandy's friend, an outside physician, told the family how important it was for Sandy to get protein and nourishment so he could heal. This is a basic tenet of postoperative healing, yet Sandy's medical team didn't concern themselves with it. The family expressed doubts and the team assuaged them, reassuring them that Sandy would start eating again soon. Pavarotti's surgeon went on a weeklong vacation, and by the time he came back and realized the gravity of the malnutrition and ordered a feeding tube, Sandy had deteriorated past the point of recovery.

Here is an example of a well-executed, lifesaving surgery that failed a patient in part because of poor aftercare — a reminder that once through the surgery, the need to advocate and keep an eye on things doesn't end.

Below are the pillars of a good surgical recovery, and things to consider as you advocate for yourself or someone else post-op.

Nutrition

As with Sandy, nutrition after surgery is highly important, its power underestimated! Protein helps with wound healing, vitamin C has antioxidant properties to protect cells from inflammatory damage, and B12 and iron are essential precursors to regenerating blood cells. Fiber and probiotics help the gut get back in gear. More on food to come soon.

Moderate Exercise

Physical therapy may commence as soon as the day after surgery. You won't be doing lunges across the room, but even slight muscle and joint activity is important to get blood moving around, stimulate the GI tract, and reorient you.

Blood Clot Prevention

Getting moving is also key in preventing deep vein thrombosis (DVT). After surgery, the blood goes through a series of changes, with a higher potential to form clots (which makes sense, as your body doesn't want you to bleed out). These conditions, however, can last up to twelve weeks after surgery. When you're relatively immobile, shored up in bed, your blood moves around less, increasing the chance a clot will form. If it breaks off and travels to the lungs, a serious or life-threatening problem called a pulmonary embolism could occur. For this reason, get moving as soon as you can, wear those terribly annoying compression stocking contraptions when you're asked to, and always alert someone if you notice a sudden change in breathing.

Pain

Severe, prolonged, improperly addressed pain will negatively impact the healing process. Stay on top of your pain, using the several tools and recommendations throughout this book to communicate with your

care team about keeping it at a tolerable
level.

■ ■ ■ ■

PART VII
WHEN YOU'RE IN
THE HOSPITAL

■ ■ ■ ■

EIGHTEEN:
BRING YOUR OWN PILLOW

Hospitals aren't terribly cozy. Their fluorescent pallor, slick floors, and uniform beds are designed with efficiency and hygiene in mind, not a good night's sleep. Add the din of conversations outside the door, intermittent beeping, and subarctic temperatures, and it's easy to feel a thousand miles from home.

This means patients should indulge and be luxurious in whatever small ways they can manage. You'll need to get creative here, and pack things that bring you comfort. They'll make for a more cozy, entertaining, and safe hospital stay, should you have to check in for a period of time to recover.

Below is a list of items to consider tucking in your bag, or sending hovering relatives off to collect:

Your favorite pillow (or two or three)
Good headphones

Soft wool socks

Something that smells like home

Essential oils

A handful of books (not only to last you, but because when you have them out the room feels a little more like a den)

A device with your music

A book on tape (many libraries offer a selection of audiobooks you can download online for free without waiting to check them out)

Your own toiletries

Your own PJs and a good robe

Loose, warm clothing

Ambient lights (like a reading lamp)

Down comforter, blanket, or quilt

Earplugs

A laptop and/or other devices as well as their chargers

ELEVATED HOMEOSTASIS

First we eat, then we do everything else.
— M. F. K. FISHER

A Word on Food

I'm with M. F. K. Fisher on this one: Food is one of the purest delights, and because delight can be in short supply during a hospital stay, I support finding ways to indulge in simple pleasures where you can. After his leg surgery, writer and neurologist Oliver Sacks invited his best friends to his room for toast and a cold split of champagne. You don't have to go grand (though you can), but it's a good idea to bring favorite shelf-stable snacks, and if you need refrigeration ask your nursing team if there is room available on the unit for you to store a few things. This is usually easy to accommodate.

Of course, depending on your condition, not everything is fair game. Your provider may tell you which foods to avoid during your healing period; the hospital also has dieticians available for consultations. If you'd like more specific advice on the best foods to eat during recovery, ask your provider or nurse to schedule a visit with one for you.

Sleep

During a hospital stay, sleep, like nutrition, is compromised at a time it's most needed. If you're struggling to get adequate rest, aside from making your quarters as luxe as possible with things from home, strategize with your nurse. They will be your champion in this regard, and often have ways to support you that you might not think of. They can, for instance:

Put a sign on your door that reroutes visitors coming to poke and prod, get you up for physical therapy, or take your dinner order, telling them to come back later.

Play bad cop and send off visitors you might not have the heart or willpower to turn away.

Cluster your care, grouping as much as possible together at one time to reduce interruptions, rather than coming in several times over the night with scheduled medications or to assess vitals.

Advocate on your behalf if you truly need to be moved to a quieter end of the unit. Nursing staff have the most sway in these decisions and can go to bat to make it happen.

COMPOSITION BOOK

Bring a notebook along for hospital stays of all lengths and levels of intensity. Keep it out where it's easily accessible so you can jot down questions as they arise. Keep track of each day and record major events, including:

Tests
Dressing changes
Visits from physical, occupational, or
speech therapists
New diagnoses
Major changes in status or direction of
care
New medications

This will help you remember what happened, and when — which can assist you in conversations with the medical team during your stay, and can also be good to have when you're going over an itemized insurance bill after the fact (see page 530, "Comb Over Your Bills"). Having your own record is a way to ensure that things are accurate.

PATIENT MENTALITY AND THE SPECTRUM OF ASSERTIVENESS

Whether you're a patient or an advocate, when you enter a modern hospital (and, for that matter, when you step into a medical encounter of any nature), leave any conditioning to be submissive at the door.

You do not get your car serviced and

think, *I hope I didn't offend them when I asked why they thought the rotation was necessary, or declined the oil change.*

It's time to assign things their proper weight. This is not an excuse to be a monster, but if there is ever a time to fight the impulse to appease authority figures and avoid making a scene, it's during your hospital stay, where it's advisable to put self-respect over respect for the system.

When I was interviewing families while working on this book, the phrase "If I could have . . ." came up consistently. Here and now, decide that you'll operate based on the assumption that (within reason) **you can.** If you want everyone in the same room, call a meeting: Tell your provider you need the specialists on your case to convene for ten minutes in your room to ensure all parties are on the same page and talking to one another. If your request is ignored, move up the chain of command (see page 381). If you're in the dark about what's going on with your diagnosis, ask questions until things make sense to you. Don't worry about how it might come across.

Hospitals will always be chaotic and busy. You will never find a nurse lying around thumbing through *Vogue*. You'll be hard-pressed to find a provider who makes you feel like they have all day to chat. The point is, if you wait for just the right moment to assert your needs, it may never come.

Don't seek conflict, but don't avoid it. If the thought of being assertive and facing collisions with practitioners and the system makes you fidget — take a moment to remember what's at stake, and weigh it objectively with the risk of stepping on toes.

Also keep in mind that the medical system is flawed — a fact lost on no one who works in the industry. Today, hospitals and clinics around the country are adopting and pro-moting cultures of transparency, meaning that clinicians are primed to admit mistakes, accept negative feedback, and address com-munication breakdowns. Reminding pa-tients about this shift in industry culture somehow reframes the dynamic and grants them permission to challenge things.

Of course, there's an art to challenging authority in a way that makes the person on the other end more receptive to your posi-tion and needs. Start from a place of align-ment rather than accusation, and you're likely to make headway. If this approach doesn't get you anywhere, your requests can take on more urgency and directness.

Though it's hard, try to remain as unemo-tional as possible in these exchanges. Amplifying a situation with tears, shouting, or attitude might be warranted, but it distracts from the issue and delays rectification.

Last, assume goodwill. Assume that your care providers have benevolence and concern for the welfare of others. Compassion and thoughtfulness are given freely. As philosopher Simone Weil would say, they are a matter of grace. Leave room for this grace to flourish, no matter how disappointed or frustrated you feel. When you look for it in the system, you'll find it.

NINETEEN:
CULTURE, CHECKS,
AND BALANCES

The following sections will walk you through how to be a patient in the hospital by introducing you to hospital culture and illustrating ways to maximize the good and mitigate the bad. Their goal is to allay common concerns as you prepare to enter the hub of the medical world.

HOSPITAL CURRENCY: THE ORDER

Think of a sheet of paper with your breakfast order, gliding along the ticket rail at a diner. Though the arrival of toast and eggs is far preferable to that of a chipper phlebotomist and their blue elastic bands, every unit of action that takes place in a hospital — from the delivery of an Alka-Seltzer to a physical therapy consult — happens through a similar, albeit more regimented, fashion.

The order is the main unit in the hospital's system of checks and balances. It ensures 1) that you, and not Jane Smith, are getting the unit of red blood cells and 2) that everyone from the pharmacist to the nurse agrees that it's the right type and that it's indicated for your condition.

At hospitals, there is a hive of activity going on around you that you can't see and a host of exchanges you aren't privy to. For example, if you're recovering from surgery and experiencing breakthrough pain, you might decide that you urgently need something stronger. Unsure when the surgeon will come by and visit on rounds (*Do I wait to ask them? Tell the nurse? Call room service?*), you settle on asking the nurse. He explains that he's used all the PRN medications available for your pain but that he will contact the surgeon to request an order for a stronger dose of Dilaudid. You hang on to your bed rails, anticipating that the process will involve a quick phone call or page — about the amount of time it takes you to bring Tylenol to your partner when they have the flu.

If the stars align, it could happen within ten minutes, but realistically it could take several hours. The order for your pain medication is not as simple as nurse-to-cabinet-to-bedside: Once the ticket is on the rail, it enters a veritable minefield of potential stalls.

Your nurse might have to tend to another acutely ill patient before they can get back to the nurses' station and put in a request to the provider. (Add twenty minutes.) When the surgeon receives the page, they might be in the middle of operating. If it's after-hours, the page might go to an on-call attending who's not familiar with your case and needs to read up before they can enter the order. (Add an hour, give or take). Once they determine it's sound to increase the Dilaudid, they enter an order into the electronic MAR (Medical Administration Record) for the new pain med, indicating dose and frequency.

From here, the order is kicked back to the pharmacist, who ensures that this new dose is appropriate and safe, given your other medications and your health status. They are a second pair of eyes to the ordering provider's. Once they approve the order, the MAR is updated to show that the new order of Dilaudid is approved. The pharmacist also has to set things in motion for the specific dose of Dilaudid to be delivered to the floor and placed in a mechanized cabinet called a Pyxis or Omnicell. This humming machine (something like the love child of a vault in Gringotts Wizarding Bank and a tarantula) talks to the electronic MAR, so when your nurse signs in with their thumb-print, the machine will alert them that the Dilaudid is approved and ready to pull. (Add another hour, give or take, from pharmacy to machine.)

Two hours and twenty minutes have now elapsed. A nurse can check the order's status at various points throughout this interval, going repeatedly to the med room to try to pull the pills, but they can't do much to speed it up.

This system is, understandably, headache inducing. *We need the Dilaudid!* But if you can grasp it, you can use it to your advantage and spare yourself as much waiting as possible.

How to Use the Order System

If you anticipate needing a medication while you're in the hospital, something over-the-counter you take at home, such as milk of magnesia or Benadryl for allergies, note them down before going to the hospital. During admission, ask the provider or nursing team to ensure they will be available to you if you need them. They will become authorized orders and available medications, even if you don't end up needing them. (See "Take as Needed: The PRN.")

If you are experiencing discomfort, especially pain, don't wait until it becomes unbearable to speak up about it. Discuss it at its earliest signs and find out what options you have to address it. (See page 259 for language to talk about pain.) Of course, you can't always anticipate discomfort, and the onset might be sudden. In these cases, remember to treat your nurse like a team member — don't channel your frustration at them. I say this because they are truly your best partner on this one, and they can and will insert themselves into the process to speed it up or sleuth out the holdup. For example, they can call the pharmacy and alert them to the order that's yet to be approved — waiting on the phone until they see the red PENDING sign disappear on the MAR in front of them.

TOO MUCH TESTING

Whenever you check into the ER or have a hospital stay, operate on the assumption that you'll get more tests than you need. You'll be poked, prodded, whisked off to radiology, and stickered up for electrocardiograms a dozen ways to Sunday. Infuriatingly, much of it may be unnecessary. Tests are often used with wild abandon, a habit that in today's medical world is born of practitioner survival. Sometimes it's done to appease insistent patients, sometimes because providers conclude the risk of missing something outweighs the time/money/risk associated with testing.

"Furor medicus" describes an intense cycle of misdirected medical activity at the patient's expense. It usually happens because a provider feels they must do something, but are unsure what. Excessive testing can fill in for substandard assessment and diagnostic skills, and providers operating within a frantic, inefficient system often have to resort to this practice.

In a system that's created the eight- to ten-minute appointment, tests are a way to ensure a better standard of care when providers can't take the time to collect a proper history, look at the case holistically, and pursue all avenues to make a proper diagnosis. Excessive testing is also a $200 billion peril on a national scale, the fiscal waste reflected in your own medical bills.

Still, tests are essential diagnostic tools, and receiving an onslaught of them can provide a sense of comfort. It's a relief to sense that everyone is on it, ruling things out and honing in on a diagnosis. The idea of something peering into our insides to see things we can't feel is reassuring!

But testing is not a net neutral when it

comes to your health. They can prime you for anxiety, to think, *If I'm getting test A, I must have condition A.* They can also lead to overdiagnosis, or overly aggressive interventions for a disease that might never cause you problems. They can create noise around the diagnostic process, adding information that can distract from the larger picture or divert attention away to things of lesser importance. And more, they can affect your long-term health: A study by the National Cancer Institute estimated that cancer diagnoses in the United States will see an uptick from excessive CT scans alone.

Settings for Excessive Testing

Teaching hospitals can be hotbeds of excessive testing. When new students get their training wheels taken off, that learning curve is steep (it's fodder for lots of laughs in the nurses' station). They have to learn somehow, and many are excellent from the get-go, but in the meantime you're their guinea pig.

Next, each time you go to the ER, you're signing up for an extensive and wide-reaching battery of tests. Be as specific as possible about your symptoms, and be extra inquisitive about the necessity of X-rays and scans they'd like to run. This is particularly true for abdominal pain of unknown origin, the most common complaint that brings people into this setting.

When you're admitted to the hospital, namely for a procedure, providers often order a standard set of tests. They might even be automatically generated orders. This is the time to talk with your providers and ensure that each test is absolutely necessary. If you just had an electrocardiogram (EKG) at an outpatient clinic the week prior, is another one necessary? If you had X-rays taken last month, can they call your PCP and request them? Go over each test and ask these questions, as paying for something unnecessary or exposing yourself to radiation twice just as a matter of policy is wasteful and detrimental. Before any test, ask:

Do I definitely need it?
Are there safer options?
How much will it cost?
What are the risks?
How will it impact things if I don't do it?

Choosing Wisely (http://www.choosing wisely.org), a campaign started for patients by the American Board of Internal Medicine, has information about overused and harmful tests and treatments. It's my best resource for determining the necessity of any given test, and I recommend it to friends and family. The site provides recommendations on tests and treatments to avoid for dozens of acute and chronic conditions, and advises on situations in which you should ask more questions before proceeding.

CHAIN OF COMMAND

There are multiple entry points to the chain of command in a medical setting, and you should choose based on the nature of the situation you need resolved. For instance, contacting a provider to inform them of poor nursing care might seem logical, but other staff can address this issue with more immediacy. Below are select links in the chain of command that will be most useful during hospital stays.

Charge Nurse

A charge nurse is responsible for overseeing care and staffing for a given shift, assigning nurses to patients, and keeping watch over the general flow of the unit. Your assigned nurse will be your number one, but you should turn to the charge nurse for issues impacting your stay outside of direct nursing care, such as a request to switch rooms, or a request to work with the same nurse when they return.

House Supervisor

House supervisors are administrative leaders who oversee the general flow of departments and entire hospitals. They sometimes run the ship during off hours, weekends, and holidays. They are the go-to source for an issue between the ER and the hospital — if you're trying to transfer, be admitted, or be released from the hospital when no one is available to help and you're running into red tape.

Nurse Manager

Nurse managers staff and manage different units in the hospital, ensuring quality of nursing care, adequate staffing, and effective policy for handling issues on the unit. Turn to one if your issue is ongoing and relates to quality of care or communication issues.

Attending Physician

Attending physicians are at the top of the hierarchy of medical professionals who come in and out of your room. You may not have one directly assigned to your case, but every resident reports to an attending, so this is where to turn if you have an issue with your provider and your provider is a resident.

Ombudsman or Patient Rights Advocate

If the above sources fail you or you're dealing with an ethical issue, call the hospital's ombudsman or patient rights advocate. They'll help you navigate the issue and provide other resources.

TAKE AS NEEDED: THE PRN

Hospital-speak is rife with acronyms, and it's easy to give up trying to decode them, but there's one important one that every hospital patient should know: PRN.

In Latin — the matriarch of medical language — *pro re nata* (PRN) means "as the thing is needed." In the context of medical care, it means there's a host of medications the provider has ordered to have on hand for you if symptoms arise. PRNs exist to control anything that might bring you discomfort during the hospital stay: pain, nausea, anxiety, GI distress, or insomnia, to name a few.

Effective PRN use depends on communication with your nurse, who can dispense them at select intervals (for example, every six hours) to stay on top of your symptoms. Because these medications are not scheduled, they depend on you speaking up. Let your nurse know when a symptom is causing you discomfort. Let your provider know if there's a medication you take from time to time at home (melatonin, Prilosec) that you'd like to have available to you. There's no such thing as "over the counter" in a hospital. The team needs to know about anything you're taking because it could interact negatively with something they're prescribing.

BEDSIDE REPORT

For the best hospital stay, it's important to understand how shifts work, especially nursing shifts. With few exceptions, shifts are usually twelve hours; 7 a.m. and 7 p.m. mark transitional periods when the floor's contained little universe is handed over to a new round of staff. The charge nurse will be replaced, and each staff nurse will hand their patients over to someone new in a ritual called the hand-off report. Practiced effectively, the hand-off report is a chance for three parties (the patient, the departing nurse, and the incoming nurse) to get on the same page, review relevant changes or significant issues, and outline the plan for the next twelve hours.

On a bad day or a less organized unit, however, the hand-off report can devolve into kvetching outside the patient's door — about their bad attitude, indolent provider, or insufferable family member. Nursing, like most medical professions, exacts a specific toll. The stress has to be metabolized — sometimes via collective commiseration after a long day (we *all* do this, no matter our occupation!) — but it shouldn't preclude the hand-off report, which research consistently demonstrates is one of the most critical processes in patient care.

An effective transition can support patient safety and reduce medical error. It's an essential part of your hospital stay, and you should request that it happen at your bedside and/or in the presence of an advocate. At the beginning of your stay, indicate that you would like to touch base with nurses during hand-off reports. Use these as an opportunity to get a sense of the twelve hours ahead and to locate yourself in the universe that will be rotating at full speed around your hospital bed.

BE A GOOD AND
MEMORABLE HUMAN

Be yourself. The world worships the original.

— INGRID BERGMAN

When you're forced to be in the hospital for any period of time, your world becomes small. It atrophies in a literal sense, as it becomes confined to the four corners of a room, and the circumstances can invite you to shut down and be passive. Amid the narrowing, however, patients also talk about the ways their world expands during this time. Where it shrinks in navigable space, it grows in other, unexpected ways.

During this time you can become a shell of your former self, or you can hold court — and I recommend the latter.

Your individuality gets whittled down from the time you're admitted. You hand over your clothes and valuables. You get into a bed, in a room identical to all the other rooms on the floor, and it's possible that slowly you become distinguishable from their inhabitants only by diseases and symptoms.

Here, the power of narrative discussed in chapter 7, "How to Talk to Providers," is at play again. Share stories when they're relevant, introduce family and friends when staff come and go, add to conversations information that gives you context, and allude to the people, places, and things outside the hospital that give your life meaning.

Put photos up. If you love to cook, write down favorite recipes to share. If you're a gardener, brag about your tomatoes! If you love reading, recommend a favorite book or pass on one you've just finished.

These small acts might seem indulgent or out of place in the medical setting. This isn't *How to Win Friends and Influence People,* after all. But these things make you human — they're a vessel for relating and the scaffolding for empathy. If nothing else, they preserve a space for human connection, a commodity in short supply in the world of modern medicine, where we don't slow down enough to let it come about organically.

BEFORE YOU LEAVE

Nothing incites cheer like hearing the word "discharge" after an extended hospital stay. You might be in such a rush toward the double doors, your dog, and your own bed that when the team comes in to discharge you, you toss the paperwork in your bag and don't look back.

We don't blame you — especially after the trials of patience we put you through in the time between sharing the happy news and then getting everything done on our end before we can actually let you leave. It's proper torture to do this to patients!

Being antsy and excited is not the best state in which to properly plan your discharge. It's like trying to listen to the teacher two minutes before class ends, or attempting to do your best work the afternoon before a vacation. It's not the best time to think of questions. It's easy to think, *I can call about that if it comes up,* and even easier to think this when you're repeatedly told during discharge, *Just call if this comes up.*

I propose going about discharges in a new way. Early in your stay, talk to friends or family about anything you're concerned may be an obstacle to recovering. Nervous about the stairs in your house? Concerned about how you'll get refills on medications prescribed in the hospital? Want to know if your insurance will continue to cover physical therapy?

Once you have a list, ask to meet with the hospital social worker or case manager. Do this early in your stay, to address your concerns and ensure that your transition out of the hospital will be as smooth as possible. If you schedule ahead, you can have your advocate present at this meeting.

Consider the following topics and prompts to come up with questions relevant to you:

What kinds of bills should you expect?

Will you have follow-up appointments? Can you get to them?

Picture a full twenty-four hours of your day-to-day routine. Will anything be newly difficult?

Do you have concerns about anything going wrong or unmanaged at home? What are they?

Do you need support services, such as occupational therapy or home health? If so, who will coordinate these services — you or the hospital?

TWENTY:
HOW TO BE VIGILANT

STORM OF ERRORS

Over a decade ago, following his fifteenth birthday, Lewis Blackman and his parents checked into a South Carolina hospital for a routine elective procedure to correct a congenital malformation called pectus excavatum, a concave sternum.

After a successful surgery on Thursday morning, problems began to arise. Lewis's IV drip was too low, leaving him dehydrated until a seasoned nurse noticed the problem and got the order changed for more fluids. By the time the fluids were fixed, it was Friday. Lewis was receiving an epidural with narcotics and a very strong form of an NSAID (in the ibuprofen family), ketorolac, via IV. By Sunday morning, it became clear that something was gravely wrong, as Lewis had a breakthrough of excruciating pain in his abdomen.

Lewis's mother, Helen, remembers a

nurse coming in and telling the family it was likely stomach pain from constipation, a common side effect of the opioids he was taking for pain. The rest of the medical team aligned with her hypothesis.

His parents tried to contact the attending doctors working on his case, but it was the weekend and they were detained at every move. The only doctor they saw was a general surgery intern, who apparently had no supervision in the hospital. Meanwhile, Lewis deteriorated rapidly over the course of the next thirty hours. By Sunday he was displaying signs of sepsis (an infection that's made its way into the bloodstream) and severe dehydration, and he was starting to exhibit signs of shock. There was still no attending to be found, staffing was low, and the family received no help in contacting the surgeon. At Helen's insistence, a senior resident from outside the hospital came, only to confirm the intern's diagnosis.

When I say Lewis deteriorated, I don't mean he exhibited subtle signs of distress or infection. The next morning, someone came in to take his blood pressure and discovered he did not have any. Convinced it was a faulty machine, they took it twelve more times using seven different cuffs, all coming up blank. They went to draw blood and couldn't, as the patient was too dehydrated and his veins had collapsed.

Within hours, Lewis died. *Mom, it's going black,* he told Helen, and she watched him arc into cardiac arrest.

Whether it came from pride, fear, or incompetence, it was a perfect storm of failure by the medical team that weekend. Lewis's death was not the result of surgery, or even complications. It was the result of communication failure, failure to escalate, failure to rescue, and lack of situational awareness.

An autopsy showed that Lewis had died from a perforated ulcer, a well-known side effect of the ketorolac he was taking. The ulcer, left unaddressed, had caused peritonitis, a deadly abdominal infection, and had eroded into the underlying artery, causing him to bleed out from the inside. A routine blood test could have confirmed the presence of infection and blood loss, but the team did not think to order it and dug their heels in as things got progressively worse.

In the years following her son's death, Helen channeled her grief into activism, getting legislation passed ensuring that patients and family members have access to an emergency response system, and that hospital staff wear badges indicating their credentials so patients always know who they're communicating with. She has altered hospital culture in a profound way. Medical and nursing students around the country are trained differently based on her recommendations, and her work has carved out new lines of communication in hospital settings, giving patients and advocates additional options for seeking help when the original team fails to hear them. I'm still learning from Helen Haskell.

During one of our recent conversations, I asked her what she does now when she or a family member enters the hospital. Her insights have shaped the following section, which reiterates that advocates and family members provide an essential safety net for patients.

MEDICATION SAFETY

To err is human. Human systems — whether they market services, orchestrate financial exchange, or govern a country — are inherently fallible because they are run by people. People who on some days show up to work with a dying relative on their mind or are suffering from a poor night's sleep. They might carry indignation toward a boss, or are intimidated and don't speak up when they notice a problem.

What sets the healthcare industry apart when it comes to flawed systems? Little, except the cost in life.

Medication error is one of the most common medical errors. Its sources, according to the World Health Organization, include:

- Lack of therapeutic training
- Inadequate knowledge of the patient's history
- Overwork and fatigue among healthcare professionals
- Poor communication among healthcare professionals and patients
- Patient characteristics (e.g., personality, literacy, language barriers)
- Complexity of the clinical case (e.g., interplay of multiple health conditions)

On page 373, "Hospital Currency: The Order," I talk about the production line revolving around a medication order. From the provider's lips to your mouth (or IV line), a medication order travels along a streamlined route, getting the seal of approval from various individuals. At each juncture, there's an opportunity for error you cannot control, but before the medication gets to you, you have a chance to safeguard yourself against nine out of ten medication errors.

While maintaining a steady belief in your hospital team's ability to care for you, recall a not-so-good day you had recently, in which you changed bags and forgot your wallet, or were distracted by a personal problem and made an error. Believe in your team, and grant them the ability to be human. Ultimately, be an active party in helping them.

Nurses are the ones who execute orders, so they are the last line of defense between you and a medication error. Each time nurses administer a medication, they verify several *right*s. Using the same model, you can be an active recipient of medications and guard against error as well:

Right patient: Ensure that the nurse verifies your first and last name and birthdate, especially if it's a new nurse you aren't familiar with.

Right medication: Ask what the medication is, and request that the pill packages be opened at your bedside. You can explain that you want to be familiar with the meds and educate yourself. Make sure it's what the provider told you they would be starting you on, or something you've been taking regularly.

Right indication: Ask why you are taking the medication. A simple "What is this one for?" will work.

Right dose: If you've been taking the medication outside the hospital: Is the dose the same? If it's a new medication, is it the typical dose for a person in your shoes?

Right time: Ask (and write down) how many times a day you will be getting the medication and when you will take it next.

Right route: If you're used to taking something orally and it's been switched to IV or a transdermal patch, inquire why. Each morning, ask for a copy of your Medical Administration Record (call it the "MAR"). Have it printed out for you in advance of each shift change, and keep it at your bedside. This printout will show you exactly what your medical team sees — your scheduled medications and what PRNs (see page 383) are available to you.

Insulin

Ask any nurse what medication they get the most safety training on, and they'll say insulin.

It's estimated that one hundred million adults in the United States have diabetes, and roughly a third of them take insulin. It's a household name, not a sexy Schedule V drug, its use so mainstream we tend to think of it as harmless. But if given in the wrong dose, insulin can be fatal. Too much can cause blood sugar to dip so low it leads to an irreversible coma or death.

So why do we let adults and children self-administer it in offices, on playgrounds, and at home? Because managing your own insulin is relatively easy once you get the hang of it. Paradoxically, the danger lies in hospital settings, where these days it's not uncommon for nurses to have several patients with diabetes on any given floor during any given shift. This means different types of the drug are given to different patients, in different doses, at different times every day. Doses depend on blood sugar, so they require recalibration each time they're administered. This translates to countless (and understandable) opportunities for error, even for the most disciplined nurse. Hospitals have systems to safeguard against these errors — nurses must verify the patient, their blood sugar, and the intended dose and type of insulin with another nurse, who must sign off before the drug is administered every time.

Still, if you take insulin you should be actively involved when it comes time to receive it in the hospital. Ask what your blood sugar is when it's taken, verify the dose and type of insulin (long-acting, fast-acting) you're receiving before every meal, and alert someone if you have any symptoms of low blood sugar (see page 309).

KEEP AN EYE ON VITALS

Nurses and physicians record vital signs and observe trends and changes to make sure things stay within defined limits. Outside of those limits, certain vital-sign ranges forewarn of a problem and are categorized via a Modified Early Warning Score, or MEWS, table.

If you had a major surgery with high risk of complication or if you've entered the hospital already compromised from other health conditions (if you have cancer, are immunocompromised, or have a chronic illness), copy down your vital signs as they are taken. It's tedious, but helpful. Keeping an extra set of eyes on that stove will never hurt. Compare your vital signs against the chart on pp. 400–401, and alert someone immediately if they enter MEWS territory.

NOSOCOMIAL NIGHTMARES

From the surgical amphitheaters of the seventeenth century to the cots and ether of the Civil War era (before germ theory and sterile technique were established!), hospitals have always been breeding grounds for microbes and disease. This means your hospitalization could come with a side of *Clostridium difficile* or MRSA. Approximately one hundred thousand people die from hospital-acquired infections every year in the United States. This section will ensure you don't become one of those statistics!

The most commonly acquired hospital infections include:

Pneumonia
GI illnesses
Urinary tract infections (UTIs)
Sepsis (an infection in the bloodstream)
Surgical-site infections

The US federal government collects and publishes data on rates of hospital-acquired infections because they impact Medicaid reimbursement. Twenty-six states also have

	3	2	1	0	1	2	3
Respirations per minute	More than 30	21–29	15–20	9–14		Less than 8	
Heart rate per minute	More than 129	111–129	101–110	51–100	45–50	Less than 40	
Systolic blood pressure (the top #)		More than 200		101–199	81–100	71–80	Less than 70

Level of consciousness	Unresponsive	Responds to pain	Responds to voice	Alert	New agitation or confusion	
Temperature		Less than 35°C	35.1–36°C	36.1–38°C	38.1–38.5°C	More than 38.6°C
Hourly urine output	Less than 10 mLs/hr	Less than 30 mLs/hr	Less than 45 mLs/hr			

*With a score of 5–6 someone on the care team should be monitoring the patient and assessing vitals every four hours.

*With a score of 7 or more, the providing care team should be called to come assess, or rapid response response should be called.

laws requiring hospitals to publicly disclose their infection rates. Those statistics can be found on the Association for Professionals in Infection Control and Epidemiology website, http://www.apic.org. With a quick Internet search, you can get the rundown on a hospital and make an informed decision on whether to proceed with surgery or a stay there.

To protect yourself from infection once in the hospital, make sure:

> That every human going in and out of your room practices scrupulous hand hygiene
>
> That before anyone uses a stethoscope or takes your vitals with a machine, it is swabbed down with alcohol in front of you
>
> To bring your own bleach wipes (and be sure to scrub, because some bacteria are feisty)
>
> That catheters aren't left in for longer than three days, and that central lines are consistently monitored for infection (see page 404 on CAUTIs, catheter-associated UTIs)

Be type A. Be brazen. The above are standard practice, but *no one* is perfect, and a good healthcare professional will never fault you for advocating for yourself in this way.

Lastly, risk of hospital-acquired infection increases the longer you're in the hospital, so don't malinger if you can help it!

Did You Wash Your Hands?

When I was in nursing school, we had a day-long lecture on handwashing: the water temp (warm), the proper sudsing method (extra attention to cuticles), how much foaming hand sanitizer one should dispense (a golf-ball-size dollop), and the frequency (over one hundred times a shift on a busy unit). We even got pointers on how to approach superiors who didn't wash their hands upon entering a patient's room.

Why all this talk about something we learn in elementary school? Because it is the number-one method of infection prevention in healthcare settings. It's so important that handwashing statistics are monitored by little hospital spies (truly!) and calculated so the public can look them up online.

Always speak up and ask the person entering your room to wash their hands if you don't witness it. You're not making a scene or being rude when you remind someone!

Lines, Drains, and Tubes Are Sources of Infection

CAUTI and CLABSI. These acronyms sound too adorable for what they stand for: catheter-associated urinary tract infection and central-line-associated bloodstream infection. Both are hospital-acquired infections that come from bacterial contamination.

For every line, drain, and tube attached to or coming out of your body, there's an increased risk of infection. This is especially true of catheters that go into the bladder and central lines that go into large veins.

Urinary catheters have to travel a considerable distance, from the outside world through genital territory, up the urethra to the bladder. They invade areas replete with microbial flora and fauna, bacteria that, if they shimmy into the wrong part of your urinary tract, can raise hell. If you or a patient you're advocating for is up for catheter insertion, do the following:

Inquire about the need for a catheter, and be sure the reason is satisfactory. If you feel that a catheter is being placed because it would take considerable staff, time, and/or care to get the patient to the bathroom and the hospital staff is trying to make it easier on themselves, push back (a lousy prehistoric practice, it's unfortunately not yet extinct).

Be sure that the person(s) inserting the catheter has washed their hands in the room before they commence, and that they don sterile gloves.

Each day, ask if the catheter is still necessary and when it will be removed. A catheter should never be left in longer than a few days. Like with houseguests and fish, things start to go south at this point.

With other intravenous (IV) lines, drains, or tubes attached to you, keep an eye on the site and alert your nurse if you notice any redness, pain, or sign of infection. They will also be monitoring for this, but it's good to have many eyes.

Call In an Infectious-Disease Specialist if You're Worried

If you're concerned about an infection in the hospital, whether it's a growing black dot that sets off necrotizing fasciitis alarms or a newly spiked fever you don't feel has gotten its due diligence — and you're not getting a satisfactory explanation or plan of action from your care team — ask that an infectious-disease specialist come to the room and give an evaluation. Most care providers have your best interests in mind, but the source of hospital-acquired infections can reflect medical error or negligence. This means that a direct member of your care team might fail to escalate this concern. Because hospital infections can create serious problems when not swiftly handled, calling a specialist is within your rights.

WRONG-SITE, WRONG-PROCEDURE, WRONG-PATIENT ERRORS

Few medical errors are as terrifying as surgery on the wrong body part or patient. While it sounds like slapstick material for a sitcom, it's common enough that it has an acronym in the medical world: WSPE.

These events are altogether rare, but they are more common than the average patient would guess. They are — understandably but inexcusably — underreported. Approximately seven occur every day in the United States.[1] While they occur across all specialties, these "never events" (as in, "should never happen") are most prevalent in orthopedic and dental contexts.

To address the sources of these errors,

regulatory boards have put policies in place such as "Sign Your Site" (which entails marking the surgical site) and presurgery "time-outs," during which the medical team stops and, one last time, verifies the patient, site, and procedure. These might sound like kindergarten activities, but they are safeguards. When the time comes to go under, the surgeon and anesthesiologist will meet with you in pre-op, where it's good practice to ask: "One last thing — for my own peace of mind, can you please verify the procedure and the site of the operation?"

WHEN NO ONE IS LISTENING

Because this book is about patient advocacy, it must cover the ways it can be thwarted in hospital settings. Below are avenues you can turn to when you've voiced a concern to the direct care team but it isn't being addressed efficiently.

Rapid response: The rapid-response team is an amazing resource. Consisting of interdisciplinary professionals (doctors, nurses, respiratory therapists), this mobile team floats the hospital and can be called to see patients on any unit. Rapid-response teams are versed in recognizing early signs of deterioration

407

in a hospitalized patient and intervening as necessary. This resource is available to clinicians, patients, and family members, so if you have concerns as a patient or an advocate, you have agency to call this team in yourself. Their number should be visible within the hospital room or posted throughout the hospital. If it's not, you can ask any staff member to share it with you.

Ethics committee: For issues of an ethical nature, this resource is available to patients and all hospital staff 24/7. You can ask for direct contact information at any time during your stay, or simply call the hospital operator and ask to be transferred.

For other concerns, reference "Chain of Command," page 381.

■ ■ ■ ■

PART VIII
WHEN YOU'RE NOT
THE PATIENT:
FAMILY MEMBERS,
PARTNERS, AND
FRIENDS

■ ■ ■ ■

Twenty-One:
You Define Family

When one of your people is thrust into the world of modern medicine — whether you're standing at a friend or partner's side as an unanticipated emergency unfolds or accompanying a family member from one appointment to the next — your role is distinct, and it is indispensable.

The following sections will support you in this role, pointing out your rights and showing how you can help the patient and their care team in ways you might not have considered.

THE PATIENT'S RIGHTS

I'll never forget a couple I once worked with on an oncology floor. The patient's partner would use the pronoun "we" when providing history and medical information to the staff. *We started the treatment five years ago. We tried the surgery, but it was ineffective.* Maybe it sounds like she was appropriating

411

her partner's pain, but at the end of the day I found it touching. She was as much our patient as he was; their experiences were bound up.

They say it most often in pediatrics, but it's true in every specialty: The patient is never just the patient. Shepherding, reassuring, and collaborating with family members are essential parts of any nurse or provider's job.

I cringe at the thought of someone being denied access to information about their partner's condition because they aren't married, or at the thought of friends intimately involved in a patient's life being dismissed by the care team because they aren't family in the strict sense of the word. Fortunately, the concept of a nuclear family is becoming obsolete as it relates to caring for the modern patient. Support systems are as diverse as the people they serve, and many care providers now recognize that. The patient defines their family, and providers should follow their lead. As a patient, you are in control of the people looped into your hospital stay, allowed in your room, and updated about your condition.

To make sure your loved ones and support network have access to you and any updates about your condition, ask for a

release-of-information (ROI) form when you are admitted, or beforehand, if it's a planned procedure. You'll be able to list the names, relationships, and contact information for anyone you'd like involved in your care. This ensures they can get information about your status and can get to you easily if they call the hospital or arrive on the unit.

HOW TO GET UPDATES IN THE HOSPITAL

My grandfather was the epitome of an avoidant patient. Up until ninety-two years of age he was still traveling and working, with only a minor health problem here and there. But one day, many years before I became a nurse, he got into bed and didn't get out for two weeks. My grandmother called to tell me he had a softball-sized tumor in his armpit and was refusing to let her or a doctor look at it. A thousand miles away and in the midst of finals, I insisted he get it looked at. Immediately. At first I pleaded calmly and rationally, then, overwrought, I flew to California. When I finally arrived at their doorstep two days later, my grandmother and I dragged him to the Scripps emergency department ourselves.

Soon I had the relief of many eyes (residents, attendings, nurses) on him, but not a clue as to the diagnosis or the treatment plan. It was complicated — it's not every day someone lets a tumor grow to the size of a softball when no one is looking. *Where are all the doctors from* Grey's Anatomy, *going to great lengths to grant his dying wishes and soak up his sage wisdom?* I wondered. *Rounds,* a friend texted. *You have to be there for the team rounds. It's the only way to get an update.* Rounds — when surgeons, providers, or teams of residents and attendings visit their patients — happen once per day in a hospital setting.

I waited patiently. I read books by his bed — leaving only to pee and grab boxed salads from the cafeteria. It was, of course, during one of these ten-minute absences that I missed rounds. My grandfather was there, but he was on morphine and as good as drunk. I planned my next day around the team's visit, but they came hours later than the day before, after I'd already gone home for the night. It took me four days to find out that he had a severely infected hair follicle (and completely unrelated Stage 4 bladder cancer).

The moral of this story? If you don't understand hospital culture, it's easy to be left in the dark when a friend, partner, or family member is in the hospital. If you find yourself in this situation, your first and best option is to go to the nurse. They will not be able to disclose test results or a diagnosis if the provider hasn't been in to see you, but they will certainly have insight. Ask them what tests have been run, what specialists are on the case, and what the plan is for the day ahead. Also ask for a general time frame for when the team will do rounds on the floor that day — they should be able to predict a one- to two-hour window. If you miss rounds, ask the nurse if they can be there, then call the unit later in the evening. By this time, the nurse will have access to new information and can share it with you.

Be sure the patient has signed a release-of-information form for you, and always call the unit before 6:30 p.m. The change of shift happens at 7, and it's nearly impossible to reach the day nurse after that, while they finish up pressing tasks. Calling after 8 p.m. will get you through to another nurse, but they may be less familiar with the case.

Provide a Baseline

In providing details about a patient's baseline, advocates can help paint a picture that healthcare providers rarely get access to. More than contextual clues that guide diagnosis, establishing a baseline allows the provider to better understand what's normal for their patient. Providers are all about trends, or how a person compares to themselves. If a patient's blood pressure usually runs low compared to the norm, we are less concerned than if we get one very low blood pressure reading during a week of relatively normal vital signs.

It helps immensely when we familiarize ourselves with trends and patterns in a patient's day-to-day life in their homes and out in the world. This is where family members, friends, and significant others can step in and dramatically change the course of care.

You are uniquely qualified to communicate your loved one's baseline to the care team. This can include their mental status, their pain, or their ability to complete activities of daily life. When the information is delivered human-to-human, the story carries more weight, sticks with providers more easily, and ensures that the fulcrum of care is the patient themselves and not statistics. Always make a point of giving a clear picture of the patient's baseline if they cannot do it themselves.

RESOURCES FOR CAREGIVERS

The universe doesn't ask your permission or review your qualifications before appointing you as someone's caregiver. Whether you assume the role as an act of unconditional love, out of familial obligation, or because there's simply no alternative — there's a point at which your reserves of benevolence, patience, goodwill, and sanity may run dry.

"You can't care for others unless you care for yourself." Nurses hear this a lot, and it irks me a little. It's objectively true, but sometimes it feels downright accusatory, a way to place the onus of responsibility on a person who is already bearing the brunt of responsibility. It's a coach standing on the hill shouting while Sisyphus rolls the stone up.

But the remark exists for a reason. Nursing has taught me to think of it more as an equation, one that reads: If I stop taking care of myself to take care of someone else, eventually I will not be around to do either. Two lives will be sacrificed (figuratively) to a disease, as opposed to one.

We are conditioned to assume the role of caregiver with immaculate grace and patience, good humor, and a steady disposition. Women, especially, are expected to balance the role effortlessly with other arenas of our lives. The role is glamorized in fiction, and poorly understood by anyone who hasn't done it. Just like having a disease yourself, being a caregiver is often isolating, especially when it's done outside of a profession. And there's not often space to have a breakdown in the context of someone else's plain-as-day objective distress, even if it's warranted.

As a nurse, witnessing patients and their loved ones interact each day, I've come to see the realities of this role — that it's at once connective and isolating, loving and boring, fulfilling and exhausting. It's often hard for a caregiver to recognize when they need help, to then demand that help, and to ultimately feel okay about demanding it (but they're entitled to a three-act play of falling apart, if that's what they need.)

If you hit that point while caring for someone in your life, here are some resources that might help:

AARP (http://www.aarp.org/caregiving): The organization has done a massive overhaul of its caregiving portal in recent years, and it is the most robust, helpful constellation of resources out there. It covers everything from local resources for respite care and support groups, to caregiving forums, to health recommendations specifically for caregivers.

Therapy: Just like there are therapists who specialize in chronic pain or relationships, there are therapists who are trained to work with caregivers. A questionnaire called the Modified Caregiver Strain Index, found at the National Center on Caregiving site (http://www.caregiver.org/depression-and-caregiving), can help you determine if you're approaching or at a point where therapy can help. After completing it, you can search for specialized clinicians.

TWENTY-TWO:
WHEN IT'S YOUR KID

My friends Kim and Mike have three kids under the age of ten, which means their household is never short on fun. Hanging out with this favorite trio of mine means learning something new approximately every thirty seconds — whether it's the lyrics to a *Hamilton* song or how butterflies migrate. They've been my introduction to the world of little people and, by extension, little patients.

Watching the crew one spring afternoon while their parents were traveling, they ran up to me upon my arrival and wasted no time telling me we were going to play emergency. They explained there'd just been a skiing accident on Mount Hood, and that I'd broken my leg and needed to wait for the doctor to come assess the situation. They told me to sit in the Adirondack chair out back and prop my foot up, ASAP. I did as I was told, and comedic gold ensued. The oldest marched out with a first-aid kit, his sister followed in a Red Cross disaster-relief vest, and the smallest of the bunch emerged with a walkie-talkie. *Girl broke her leg trying to do a black diamond. Over and out.*

They blew through every Band-Aid and alcohol wipe in the kit. They reset my tibia with plastic tweezers, made my bruises vanish with an ice pack, and checked in on my pain levels. They made sure someone went to the waiting room to let my parents know I would make a speedy recovery and walk again thanks to their efforts, but that I would need to stay in the hospital for about six years. They explained that even though I was hurt, I shouldn't worry because I was in the greatest hands. Determining it was a sensible time to kill two birds with one stone, they gave me a flu shot, too. They brought the dog to distract me and administered it via Q-tip. They explained everything they were going to do in detail before they did it. I was in awe.

As the scene went down, I realized that this brilliant display of pretend reflected their first encounters with the world of medicine, namely their pediatricians. They were emulating the care and attention they'd received when they were hurt or sick, or going in for a checkup. They showed me that most of what we come to know and believe about being a patient is shaped by our pediatricians.

FINDING AND WORKING
WITH A PEDIATRICIAN

Part teacher, part confidant, and part care provider, pediatricians are a category unto themselves. They support families from the time children are born through their adolescence, counseling them on significant matters of development from breastfeeding to teen substance abuse. For this reason, it's especially important to find someone your child connects with and can grow with.

All the ideas outlined in "North Star: How to Choose a Primary Care Provider" can be adapted to find a great pediatric provider, basically a PCP for little patients. Here are some good questions to ask when you're meeting them for the first time:

What is your philosophy about:
    Breastfeeding?
    Vaccinations?
    Sleep and discipline issues?
How would I reach you if I thought something was wrong?
Who covers for you when you're away?
How long does a typical checkup last?

422

Once you've found one, remember the power of questions (see "How to Talk to Providers")! During your first newborn appointment with your chosen pediatric provider, no question is crazy. This is the place to ask about everything from burping to chapped nipples.

There's a lot of overlap in the Venn diagram of pediatric care issues and general parenting issues. Pediatric providers, just like teachers, can help you address some difficult territory specific to kids, such as:

Obesity
Bullying
Internet safety
Drug and alcohol use
Smoking and tobacco use
Sexual health and sexual orientation
School violence
Stress

As your child flies through infancy into childhood and they're ready to be a more active participant, they'll begin learning how to be a patient. Here are a few things you can do to empower them:

Make a project out of sitting down with your kid and compiling their medical records. Maybe a bright-pink Lisa Frank folder is the ticket to making it a practice they'll carry into adulthood! (HIPAA, the medical privacy law, allows parents to access their young children's medical records, so as a parent you have the right to collect these just as you would for yourself. See page 128 for instructions on accessing medical records.)

Before you and your child head off for an appointment, have a conversation with them, whatever their age, about how their body is doing. They may need you to help advocate for them. On the other end of the spectrum, especially as they get older, they may want to talk to their provider without you in the room. Try to respect this autonomy.

Make sure that whoever accompanies your kid to appointments (if you can't) is equipped with information about their diet, sleep, behavior, and activity that they can relay when asked.

In interviewing patients and pediatricians, a few topics emerged consistently. The big ones — vaccination myths, infant safety issues, preparing for pediatric hospitalization, and tests and medications your child may or may not need — are addressed in the rest of this chapter.

VACCINES: MYTHS AND FACTS

Vaccines given in the first two years of life are a raindrop in the ocean of what an infant's immune system successfully encounters and manages every day.
— CHILDREN'S HOSPITAL OF PHILADELPHIA

In your earliest years of parenthood, the issues you're confronted with are of the here and now. When you're thinking about whether to pay extra for organic baby food, diphtheria feels like an ancient disease from a distant world we've left behind. So why concern yourself with vaccines? There are three critical reasons:

To prevent infections that circulate today. Many potentially fatal diseases still circulate in the United States today, including chicken pox (varicella zoster), mumps, and whooping cough (pertussis). These diseases are invisible and potentially fatal, and they aren't selective in where they emerge and who they infect. Choosing to forgo vaccination means accepting the possibility that a child will contract one of them. As pediatrician Lisa Tumarkin puts it, "I tell parents that they are making an active choice when they decide to withhold a vaccine." She's right: In 2018, 85 percent of the children who died from the flu were unvaccinated.

To prevent new outbreaks of infections. Some infections aren't common but still exist and can surface without warning. If they aren't kept at bay with vaccinations, they can spread quickly. In the late eighties, for instance, an outbreak of measles in Los Angeles cost many kids their lives. Scientists concluded that without better immunization compliance in preschool-age children, the epidemic was likely to reoccur.

To protect children in other countries. Polio and diphtheria are not threats in the United States today, but they are in other parts of the world. Children are still paralyzed by polio in Afghanistan and Nigeria and can catch diphtheria in India and other countries in Southeast Asia. When unvaccinated children travel internationally, they can cause reemergence of these outbreaks.

Confronting Conflicting Information about Vaccines

There's generally an ongoing disconnect between the information you take in about vaccines from the media and what you're told by health professionals in a pediatric office. The topic is rife with misinformation, a byproduct of the autism scandal of the late nineties.

It often puts parents at ease to know that individual pediatricians do not decide which vaccines to give out and when. Instead, they follow vaccination schedules created by a team of experts at the Centers for Disease Control and Prevention (CDC), composed of clinicians and scientists (many of them parents of young children). They sift through evidence about vaccine efficacy and safety and ensure that vaccination schedules are based on studies that are meticulously performed, reproducible, and published in peer-reviewed journals. (This means studies meet the highest criteria for reliability, and their results are corroborated by independent institutions.) Teams of fiercely dedicated individuals have devoted their careers to reading scientific literature on your behalf. Take comfort in the fact that if an alarming article appears denouncing the latest HPV vaccine or proposing to split the vaccination schedule, it won't slip by this panel.

More important facts:

Vaccines do not cause autism.

A child still needs vaccines while breastfeeding. Maternal antibodies do not provide sufficient protection.

Vaccines cannot cause the disease they are protecting a child from.

The amount of aluminum found in vaccines (approximately four thousandths of a gram) is established to be safe. The concentration is lower than that found in breast milk (and *much* lower than in infant formula) and has been shown not to impact serum levels of aluminum in infants.[1]

Though it can be daunting to think of a baby or young child getting so many shots at once, following the vaccination schedule is the safest approach. It's ill-founded to split the vaccination schedule, space it out, or withhold specific vaccines (except for reasons related to health or allergy status). Consequences of doing so range from child stress each time they have to face a needle, to infecting newborns or immunocompromised grandparents, to national outbreaks because of lapses in immunization.

To ensure you don't miss an appointment, set a reminder on your calendar for one month before your child's birthday to schedule each appointment. Just be sure the appointment is after the child has turned the age listed in the CDC pediatric vaccination schedule (see appendix).

Fear of Needles

If your child doesn't have a charged response to needles, check to make sure they're not an alien! For many of us needles cause anxiety, beginning in the early years and sometimes lasting through adulthood.

For kids, and even adults, there's an excellent helper called a ShotBlocker. It's a little plastic pad that's pokey on one side, and when it's held to the skin during a shot, it distracts the sensory nerves (and the patient) from the pain signals caused by the needle poke. Studies have shown the gadget is effective at reducing pain and distress during intramuscular injections. Florida pediatrician Lisa Tumarkin keeps them stocked in her clinic to boost courage and ease discomfort when vaccines are due, but

429

you can also purchase one yourself and bring it along to appointments with your little one.

PEDIATRIC HOSPITALIZATION

When Should I Take My Kiddo to the ER?

With a few specific exceptions, the answer here is to trust your gut. With newborns, a temperature above 100.5°F warrants immediate care. Other things that should send you on your way include a newborn who is difficult to wake up or a newborn who stops eating or peeing.

Kids with asthma should be taken to the ER if they have any signs of strenuous breathing, especially wheezing that abruptly stops. If your child has asthma, talk to your pediatric provider and make sure you understand all the warning signs that should direct you to an emergency department.

Otherwise, it's really how a kid looks. Sick kids look different to their parents. It may sound basic, but this gut feeling is a more telling indicator that something is wrong than fever, poop, or puke.

Some pediatric practices connect patients' families with twenty-four-hour access to a phone triage program to help parents determine if an ER trip is necessary. Ask your pediatric provider if they have or recommend one, and how you can access it.

Childhood Illness and Hospitalization: Resources

Many large hospitals (especially pediatric hospitals) have a department called Child Life Services, with professionals trained in easing the hospitalization process on little patients and their families (whether it's for a short procedure or long-term chronic illness management). These professionals tend to be passionately devoted to their work and are beloved among families for bringing normalcy into the hospital experience and ensuring that childhood is not sacrificed to hospital culture. They're able to explain cancer in terms a five-year-old can understand, provide emotional support to parents and children during difficult procedures, incorporate play into the patient's schedule, and orchestrate peer interactions for teens navigating long-term hospitalization. Talk with your pediatric provider to ask for contacts and resources at larger hospitals when you set the date of a procedure or stay.

RECOMMENDED READING

The following are a few award-winning books recommended by pediatricians for young children heading to the doctor or on the precipice of surgery or hospitalization. They address complicated topics and can empower young readers with knowledge and a sense of confidence when it comes to being a patient.

Shine-A-Light: The Human Body, by Carron Brown and Rachael Saunders

Kids can use a flashlight to illuminate the book's drawings and reveal a baby in utero, muscles flexing, and bones. It's a fun way to get kids interested in exploring the mysteries under their skin and asking questions about them. It can be a good starting point to learning about a body part or condition prior to a procedure.

The Surgery Book: For Kids, by Shivani Bhatia

Written by an anesthesiologist, this book is told from the perspective of a little boy named Iggy as he gets his tonsils taken out. It's a great intro to hospital culture and a starting point for discussing different kinds of surgeries and allaying common childhood fears.

Clifford Visits the Hospital, by Norman Bridwell

I might be biased because I have a big red dog, but this classic really covers all the bases, and kids love it. It's an excellent tool to prepare kids for longer hospital stays, or to help siblings and friends understand what's going on when their peer is in the hospital.

TWENTY-THREE:
WHEN YOU'RE GETTING OLDER
(OR WHEN IT'S YOUR PARENT)

SWITCHING TO A GERIATRICIAN

As this book covers health across the life-span, the information in the following sections apply if you're transitioning into old age, or caring for someone else who is. You'll find that just like pediatrics, geriatric care is a field unto itself and requires special considerations.

Elderly patients, more than any other population, need care that is suited to their individual needs and accommodates them. When it comes to diagnosis and treatment, their care needs to take into consideration the differences in symptom presentation and physiological processes that come with aging.

All providers should have a basic knowledge of geriatric medicine, but in many cases they don't have the depth of knowledge needed for specialized care. I recommend starting to think about switching to a geriatrician around age sixty-five and actually doing it by seventy, barring any complicated conditions (in which case, do it sooner). You can ask for references from your primary care provider, going through a vetting process similar to the one discussed earlier in this book (see page 70). You can also refer to http://www.healthinaging.org for a helpful tool to search for geriatric providers in your area.

QUESTIONS SPECIFIC TO OLDER ADULT PATIENTS

Older adult patients and/or their advocates should ask the following questions at every appointment or before any procedure.

At Appointments

What is being treated? Is it a syndrome or a disease?

It's not uncommon for an acute condition or malady in an elderly patient to be the result of several contributing factors, rather than a specific etiology. Providers will often treat a cluster of symptoms — a syndrome — rather than a disease. Knowing which it is can shape your understanding of the course of treatment and care.

This question is especially important in addressing confusion. Confusion can be assessed and treated with the approach that its source is dementia, or that its source is transient — a symptom of delirium or a urinary tract infection. The treating provider should clearly delineate and explain this, but in the chaos they may not. The provider may also just not know the cause, which is important information for you to have as well.

For Medications

Is a generic version of the drug available?

Has this been called into the pharmacy? When can I retrieve it?

Could this interact with any other foods or prescriptions I am/they are taking?

What medications are we adding and taking away?

For Recommended Procedures

Are there alternatives to surgery?

Can you give me a thorough explanation of the risks and benefits of this procedure?

What happens if we do nothing?

What type of anesthesia will be used?

Is there a surgeon/anesthesiologist/provider available to do the procedure who specializes in geriatric patients?

What will the recovery time be in best- and worst-case scenarios?

What will follow-up care entail — physical therapy? Skilled nursing?

TOO MANY MEDICATIONS

In elderly patients, a new illness or symptom should not be attributed to the aging process or a new disease until it's been definitively determined that it is not caused by medications. Adults over the age of sixty are especially vulnerable to the effects of polypharmacy (see page 157), which can cause falls, more frequent hospitalizations, and increased mortality. If you are the advocate for an older adult patient, keep this issue in mind. The following section has a list of medications that older adults should usually avoid taking. Question the provider further if one of them is prescribed.

Beers Criteria

The Beers Criteria is a list of medications that should be used cautiously or avoided completely with older adult patients (those sixty-five or older). It is an essential resource for health practitioners — and it can be for you as well. Created in 1991, it's reviewed by the American Geriatrics Society and updated consistently every few years as new information comes out. You can access it at http://www.geriatricscareonline.org, but for quick reference, the top medications and classes on the list are:

NSAIDs (nonsteroidal anti-inflammatory drugs) — used to treat pain
    Example: ibuprofen
Digoxin (Lanoxin) — used to treat irregular heartbeats and/or heart failure
Select diabetes medications
    Examples: glyburide (DiaBeta, Micronase), chlorpropamide (Diabinese)
Benzodiazepines
    Examples: diazepam (Valium), alprazolam (Xanax), chlordiazepoxide (Librium)

Sleeping pills
>Examples: zaleplon (Sonata), zolpidem (Ambien), eszopiclone (Lunesta)

Muscle relaxants
>Examples: cyclobenzaprine (Flexeril), methocarbamol (Robaxin), carisoprodol (Soma)

Select anticholinergics

Select antidepressants
>Examples: amitriptyline (Elavil), imipramine (Tofranil)

Trihexyphenidyl (Artane) — used to treat Parkinson's disease

Dicyclomine (Bentyl) — used to treat irritable bowel syndrome

Meperidine (Demerol) — used to treat pain

Products that contain the antihistamines diphenhydramine (Benadryl, Tylenol PM) and chlorpheniramine (Aller-Chlor, Chlor-Trimeton) — often found in OTC remedies for coughs, colds, and allergies

Haloperidol (Haldol), risperidone (Risperdal), quetiapine (Seroquel), unless the patient is being treated for psychosis — used to treat behavioral problems in older adults with dementia

Estrogen pills and patches — used to treat

hot flashes and other menopausal symptoms

SYMPTOMS IN OLDER ADULTS

If you've ever worked with older adult patients, when the day comes that Mrs. S suddenly sees an imaginary poodle in the corner of the room, your first thought is *not* Alzheimer's or schizophrenia — it's a urinary tract infection (UTI). One among many of the atypical symptoms associated with aging, a UTI-caused hallucination is an unforgettable example that with older adult patients, the habits we've acquired and the parameters we've adopted for identifying medical problems might not hold. The connection between a condition and a symptom can be different in an older adult, and a symptom that warns of an acute problem in a younger patient can be absent in an older adult patient. Confusion can indicate a UTI; infections are only rarely indicated by fever; a hyperactive thyroid may cause a patient to be slow and fatigued rather than hyperactive; and new-onset agitation can be a symptom of a slow thyroid. Heart attacks and cancers are more likely to be silent.

Keep this in mind when you're an older patient or taking care of an older patient, especially when you're keeping track of the care plan for treatments and hospitalizations.

GET THE SHINGLES VACCINE

If you've ever had shingles, you know it can be like contracting the modern-day equivalent of the bubonic plague. Shingles emerge from varicella zoster, the fancy name for the viral strain that causes chicken pox. For unknown reasons, the virus never really leaves us. After the days of quarantine and calamine lotion are through, it goes dormant, camping out in the spine until something reactivates it. The older virus re-emerges not as chicken pox but as inflammation of the nerve ganglia, which translates to pain. The ganglia serve different patches of skin, which determines where the rash appears, like shingles on a roof. Replete with blisters and searing pain, the disease also poses a threat to vision and can inflict neuropathic pain that goes on for years after the rash resolves.

The disease sounds medieval, but today adults over the age of fifty possess a sharply increased risk of contracting it. Many of us contracted chicken pox as youngsters, whether the symptoms were full-blown or inconspicuous, and studies have shown that by the time you're eighty, you have a one-in-three to one-in-two chance of getting shingles. Also note that having had shingles in the past does *not* mean you won't get it again, and you can't catch shingles from another person, but a person who has never had chicken pox (or the chicken pox vaccine) can get chicken pox from someone with shingles.

If I sound hyperbolic, it's because I'm imploring you to get vaccinated and spare yourself the misery. If you're not an older patient yourself, ensure that your parents and grandparents get the vaccine. Perhaps even more of a no-brainer than the flu shot, Shingrix, the new silver bullet of shingles vaccines, is 97 percent effective at preventing cases in adults over the age of forty and 90 percent effective at preventing cases in those over seventy.

Patients can start getting the vaccine around age sixty. It requires two separate shots two months apart and is effective for up to six years. Those who are immunocompromised (for example, from HIV or chemotherapy) are still candidates for the vaccine and should discuss it with their provider.

Because of the way Medicare and Medicaid categorize and cover the vaccine, it is currently often easiest to have it done in a pharmacy (reimbursement can be delayed if it's done in a doctor's office). By the time this book reaches you, though, it might be a walk in the park, so talk to your provider.

RECOGNIZING DELIRIUM

To experience delirium in a hospital setting can be a harrowing experience. And while it affects close to 20 percent of hospitalized adults over the age of sixty-five, the average person hasn't heard of it outside the context of delirium tremens (the DTs), the state that comes about during a withdrawal from alcohol.

Delirium is an acute change in mental status (attention, awareness, cognition) that develops over hours to days, and typically fluctuates over the course of a twenty-four-hour period. It can be triggered by a plethora of seemingly benign symptoms ranging from impaired vision and hearing to a fever. The underlying mechanisms are vast and difficult to trace and correlate.

To get an idea of what it feels like, I've heard it described as dropping a tab of acid a few days into a hospital stay. Delirium is often accompanied by hallucinations, delusions, sundowning (dysregulated sleep and wake cycles), incoherent speech, disorganized thoughts, and agitated or aberrant

443

behavior. But the symptoms can be much subtler and less pronounced, depending on the person in whom they manifest.

The following factors make someone more vulnerable to developing delirium, so be especially vigilant when they are in the hospital:

Older age
Alcoholism
Severe fever
Infection
Metabolic disturbance (acidosis)
Mechanical ventilation
Cognitive impairment (dementia)
Depression
Hypertension
Vision or hearing impairment
Heart disease
History of previous delirium

Because delirium is especially common in (but not limited to) older adults, it can be confused with dementia. To mistake it for dementia can be a grave misstep, because the underlying causes of delirium can be acutely life-threatening if not attended to. If you're an advocate, communicating information about the patient's baseline (see page 415) is crucial.

Delirium commonly occurs in hospitals because of the unfamiliar surroundings and schedule, combined with a compromised physical state, but it can also occur in community and residential settings such as skilled nursing facilities, rehabilitation centers, and nursing homes.

HOW TO DIFFERENTIATE DELIRIUM FROM EARLY-STAGE DEMENTIA

Delirium has a rapid onset, unlike dementia, which typically progresses slowly over time (unless it follows a stroke).

Alertness (ability to keep eyes open and respond to stimuli in the environment) is impaired with delirium, but not with dementia.

Patients with delirium often exhibit slurred or incoherent speech and delusional or disorganized thought patterns, while patients with dementia exhibit impoverished thoughts and have difficulty finding words.

It would be easy to chalk up any of these symptoms to old-age battiness or side effects from heavy medications given in the hospital. If any of the following scenarios are true, though, it warrants getting a provider in to assess the patient immediately:

Did the changes come on suddenly?

Do the changes come and go, with vacillating severity throughout the day and night?

Is the person having trouble paying attention to you or following what's going on, in a way that's abnormal for them?

Is the person difficult to rouse, especially lethargic, or in a stupor?

It can be torturous to watch someone go through this acute distress, not to mention traumatic for the patient. If you've recognized it and alerted someone on the medical team, their response should be immediate — an assessment should be done within thirty minutes. If it doesn't happen, you can call rapid response and get a team in yourself (see page 407).

MENTAL HEALTH SUPPORT: A CAVALRY FOR LONELINESS

One night last spring I tuned into a story on the BBC about a group of firefighters in Bellingham, Washington, who responded to an afternoon call from an elderly gentleman. "He thinks it's a heart attack," the dispatcher told them.

When the firefighters arrived, a man in suspenders answered the door and invited them inside. As the scene unfolded, the firefighters realized it was a call not of distress but of hospitality. He ushered them to the living room and offered to make tea. "Yes, my heart was pounding like an elephant was standing on me, then it stopped!" he explained, sharp and steady on his feet.

They assessed him for good measure and then, nonplussed, obliged him. The men in gear kept their radios on and stayed just shy of an hour. They talked about the football season and the low tide and told him his heart was in good shape. "We could have felt tricked," one of them recalled, "but it was easy to see ourselves answering that door someday."

There are unacceptable reasons to call 911, and of course loneliness is one of them. But I'm still smiling as I write this. This guy got away with something, and I'm all for it.

Having been raised by older adults and having worked with them as a nurse has proven to me that feeling heard, respected, dignified, and part of a larger community is essential to our ability to thrive. A reverence for this fact should be integral to care. I can put names and faces to a body of research demonstrating that older adults disproportionately experience depression. Even if you prefer to call it the blues or loneliness, it still means a compromised quality of life.

Depression is not a natural part of the aging process, and should not be minimized as such. Generational differences in feelings about mental health render it difficult to identify and treat depression in older adults. One result is that the suicide rate for white men over the age of eighty-five is six times the national average. But in most cases, the depression that precedes it is a treatable episode.

Whether you're an older adult yourself or you are advocating for a friend or family member, make sure mental health is discussed at each primary care appointment. The Geriatric Depression Scale (http://geriatrictoolkit.missouri.edu/cog/GDS _SHORT_FORM.PDF) is useful to take and discuss with a provider. Primary care providers can write prescriptions for effective medications to combat depression — and this is usually their go-to. In bypassing a referral to a psychiatric practitioner or therapist, they can spare the patient the logistics of additional appointments. Even so, I suggest following up with a licensed mental health professional in the form of regular therapy. Many practitioners who are covered by Medicare and other insurance carriers will even make house calls or visit residential care facilities — you just need to call around and ask. The Geriatric Mental Health Foundation (http://www.gmhfonline.org) is a good place to start.

Finally, those of you who are not yet elderly yourself can help by looking out for older adults within your community. Older adults tend to be wiser, kinder, more generous with their time, more honest with their advice, and more present. American society's refusal to cherish them as other cultures do is one of its great shames. I'll leave you with a sign-off from one of the last letters my grandfather wrote me, taken from a Fitzgerald novel:

At fifteen, you had the radiance of early morning
　At twenty, you will begin to have the brilliance and melancholy of the moon

And when you are my age, you will give out, as I do, the genial golden warmth of 4 p.m.

COMMUNICABLE DISEASE AND COMPROMISED IMMUNITY

Aging comes with compromised immunity. Older adult patients, particularly those with cancer or hepatitis, are especially vulnerable to nosocomial (acquired in the hospital) infections like the flu, MRSA, and *Clostridium difficile.* When you or an older adult patient you're advocating for is in the hospital, be militant about handwashing whenever anyone enters or exits the room. If a room on the unit has a sign on the door noting "PPE required" (meaning "personal protective equipment" — symbols will vary from hospital to hospital) turn the dial up on your militancy, because the person in that room has a communicable disease. It doesn't warrant a panic attack or requesting to change units, but stay on your toes.

FACTOR IN FRAILTY

Specific to older adult patients is an X factor that impacts medical decisions: frailty. While it sounds like an abstract concept, the Frailty Index for Elders (FIFE) measures it. It provides insight into a patient's medical vulnerability profile (loss of function, loss of physiological reserves) and can help predict surgical outcomes and treatment responses.

For instance, surgery might be the obvious fix for a fifty-year-old with a tumor, but for an eighty-year-old, the intervention could set off a cascade of problems that alter the risk-benefit analysis. The surgery and the extra recovery time that follows might translate to extra days in the hospital, increasing the chances of a hospital-acquired infection or a fall resulting in a fracture due to postsurgical weakness. In turn, these things could reroute the patient to a rehab or skilled nursing facility rather than home, which might instigate depression. Frailty is often a good indicator of the likelihood of these what-ifs.

Similarly, an assessment can be helpful when making decisions about aggressive cancer treatments such as chemotherapy, or even whether a patient requires more supportive care at home.

FAMILIARIZE YOURSELF WITH THE BEST TREATMENT MODELS

A number of treatment models in hospitals can be particularly helpful to elderly patients.

ACE: Inquire about Acute Care for Elders (ACE) units in hospitals. These are designed with the unique challenges of the elderly in mind.

NICHE: Nurses Improving Care for Healthsystem Elders (NICHE) is a training and certification program for nursing staff who will have the most direct care of elderly patients in a hospital setting. Certification indicates that the nurses have undergone specialized training in the unique needs and safety issues relevant to older adults.

Interdisciplinary approach: Just as with patients with a chronic illness, there are many moving parts, all equally important, when providing an older adult with comprehensive, relevant care. For this reason, an interdisciplinary approach to care is the best route. In this approach, various specialists come together around a case in a central location (rather than the case floating back and forth between them), and social workers, dieticians, pharmacists, nurses, and physical therapists are also involved. A multiperspective approach is always beneficial, especially for older patients with multiple interacting conditions, so look for clinics that operate with this model.

GETTING TO AND FROM

Transportation is often the biggest barrier to care for older adult patients, who may not be able to drive, have limited mobility, or require accommodation for a wheelchair or scooter. Below are some options that can remedy this issue. Also check your county's Senior Services or Department of the Aging website, as they list resources dedicated to helping elderly patients get to appointments.

Medical Transportation Services

There are professionals whose sole job is to transport patients, and they are experienced in mobility assistance. They help the patient from their doorstep to the waiting room and wait for the appointment to end so they can help them back again. It's almost like a hospital Lyft system! A quick online search will direct you to companies in your vicinity, and you can also call your hospital for references.

It's becoming more common, and less prohibitively expensive, to find providers who make house calls. Even health systems like Kaiser are adopting programs to make this possible for senior patients. If it would benefit you or someone you care for, factor it in as an option.

END OF LIFE

Practice dying.

— PLATO

Many doctors and surgeons I know have staunch feelings about dying in the hospital under advanced medical care — they refuse to do it. In the same vein, many oncology nurses would tell you they'd decline third and fourth rounds of chemotherapy under most circumstances. Many intensive care unit nurses would tell you they wouldn't want to be admitted to their own units, which house the most sophisticated technology in existence to extend life beyond its natural culmination.

Many of us in the industry have seen patients suffer as a result of our collective inability to shepherd them through the dying process gracefully. We want to avoid the same fate.

The literature has shown that about half of providers paint a rosier picture when relaying news about a terminal illness. This is an injustice that can gravely alter how someone lives out the end of their life. "Medicine's focus is narrow," Atul Gawande points out in his book *Being Mortal.* "Medical professionals concentrate on repair of health, not sustenance of the soul. Yet — and this is the painful paradox — we have decided that they should be the ones who largely define how we live in our waning days."

If you die in the hands of the medical system and have some agency in the process, like many of us will, there will come a point when you must decide who will make the decisions about *how* it happens: you or your medical providers. My hope is that this section will guide you in making these decisions with your team or on your own, rather than letting anyone make them for you.

Why You Might Not Get the Truth

Too few doctors, it is true, treat their patients as whole human beings, but the reverse is also true. I have always tried to be gentle with my doctors, who often have more at stake in terms of ego than I do. I may be frustrated, maddened, depressed by the incurability of my disease, but I am not diminished by it as they are. When I push myself up from my seat in the waiting room and stumble toward them, I incarnate the limitation of their powers. The least I can do is refuse to press on their tenderest spots.

— NANCY MAIRS, WRITER AND MULTIPLE SCLEROSIS PATIENT

When a patient is terminally ill and the treatment options left to pursue become a matter of quantity vs. quality of days, it challenges the very foundation of the medical model. Providers seem to unravel accordingly. You enter the world of medicine to get well, and when it's been determined you cannot, the patient-provider relationship falters. Stripped of their ability to cure, providers may shut down, avert their eyes, and pacify rather than initiate difficult conversations. Their innate aversion to this outcome and their increasing access to therapies and technologies to stave it off cause medical professionals to fail patients in their final chapters.

I once stood in the corner of the room waiting to give a medication while a surgeon came to do rounds on our patient dying of breast cancer. This typically gregarious doctor suddenly had a flat affect and couldn't look the patient in the eyes when he spoke. "Was it just me?" she asked once he left the room. "Did you notice it too?" I nodded. She was the embodiment of his limitations.

How Long Do I Have? vs. A Working Timeline

A swell of fear accompanies the initial understanding that death is near and the path forward is uncertain. It's human nature to want to know how long you have remaining. There's comfort in answers. But everyone (patients, practitioners, you, and I) needs a gentle reminder that medicine only goes so far, and that when you ask "how long?" you will receive at best an educated guess.

A working timeline is more useful — it's flexible and allows you the liberty to adjust your decisions day-to-day. Your medical team can help you establish a timeline, and they will be eager to do it. It requires a more delicate conversation, though, and you'll need to learn about the different stages and physical manifestations your illness will take as it advances. But a discussion about each of these stages can include a plan for how to accommodate symptoms as they arrive, and provide insight into what you'll be capable of physically and mentally.

It's important to decide how you want to spend your time. Let that shape your decisions about whether your priority is quality of time or quantity.

Do you want to be:
Social?
Outdoors?
Around family?
Alone?
Near water?
With your pets?
In another city or country?

Do you want to be able to:
Read and write?
Garden?
Travel?
Keep working as long as possible?

Do you feel safer:
At the hospital?
At home?

Is your biggest concern:
Pain?

Fatigue?

Confusion or cognitive impairment?

Once you've thought about some of these things, go over them with someone (or several people) you trust from your care team. It's better to have this conversation earlier. In fact, it's *never* too early to start the dialogue.

Where You Are Matters

There are certain hospitals I would not choose to die at. When I was in nursing school, I did back-to-back clinical rotations on medical oncology units. One was at a small, religiously affiliated hospital, and the other was at a world-renowned hospital. While I might go to the latter if I was in the early stages of fighting a disease, I would go to the quaint hospital to get care at the end of my life. This particular hospital had a robust palliative care team that had been working together for years. Where the quaint hospital offered a menu of services like extended visiting hours, pet therapy, and private consultations with radiant individuals with abundant experience helping people navigate the dying process, the big hospital would send in a team of white coats to talk to you about your poor prognosis. The extent of their intervention would usually be putting a sticker on the door indicating that you were transitioning to comfort measures only.

These are extremes. In any setting, your experience will be determined largely by the individuals overseeing your care and your willingness to communicate openly with them. Still, consider that the best hospital to seek treatment in and the best hospital to die in might look very different for you.

Hospice, Palliative Care, and Comfort Care

Several years ago I worked with a patient in her late eighties named Sadie, who was admitted from the hospital's emergency department up to the oncology floor. She didn't have cancer, but all the other units were full, so she ended up with us. When I arrived and received a handoff report the morning after she'd been admitted, the other nurses were in a *mood,* and soon I realized why.

Sadie was not a stranger to the hospital. She had terminal chronic obstructive pulmonary disease (COPD) and heart failure, with a poor prognosis and little time left before her organs gave out. She came to the emergency department not for her heart or breathing but because she had excruciating pain in her calves from constricted vasculature. She came because she needed relief from the pain.

Because her disease was in its final stages, Sadie was working with a palliative care team. When a patient switches over to palliative care, a team of doctors, nurses, and social workers specializing in end-of-life care oversees their case. The goal shifts from curative interventions to maximizing comfort and quality of time.

But on our floor, the providers were less familiar with her case and she was greeted by a team of first-year residents who weren't aware of her palliative care status. They withheld certain pain medications that under normal circumstances would be contraindicated (potentially harmful) for a person like Sadie, with advanced heart and lung disease. So she suffered with her leg pain until the sun came up and the palliative care team arrived on the floor to correct things and read the residents the riot act.

Sadie got her pain medication. She started telling stories and passing her favorite perfume around for the nurses to sniff. Over the next forty-eight hours, her family started to come with food and other unexpected delights. (Someone even snuck in Sadie's Pomeranian, Baby Girl, in their purse for a visit — to which I turned a blind eye because, well, I'm not a monster.) We brought every folding chair on the unit into her ten-by-ten room. There was a lot of merrymaking and storytelling, and then she died.

I think about the many universes in which this case could have gone a different way. Sadie could have been at another hospital without a strong care program, where her death, when it came, would not have reflected agency or peace. She could have been in severe pain throughout. Her medical team could have delivered news in a way that gave her hope she might last another six months. They could have told her she was dying only at this very visit, when she had a few days left rather than months.

Patients often think palliative care, comfort care, and hospice are synonymous with giving up, and worry their medical team will do the same and their care will spiral. Some worry they'll be left in a room at the end of the hall in the abandoned corners of the hospital basement. This is far from the case.

This type of care is a lateral shift, not a cessation. Rather than taking away aspects of care, it adds in new ones with a different focus. The general principle is that when someone decides to switch to specialized end-of-life care, they're afforded *more* choice and flexibility than they were before.

Because these services signify transition to the end, they're often used as a last resort, at the final hour. In most cases, though, they're accessible to patients well before that point. Patients and family members often tell me they feel like they're getting away with something once they figure out the secret — which is to use palliative care, especially hospice, as early as possible. This is because they make life infinitely easier for the patient and caregivers when it comes to getting medication, attention, and logistical support when and where it's needed. It's a significant pivot, from the *hospital* being the locus of care to the *patient* being the locus of care.

Some of the benefits to this mode of care include:

The ability to get personalized, hospital-level care at home

Access to a care team 24/7

Reduced financial burden (Medicaid, Medicare, and most private insurances cover these services)

Family support and grief counseling
Fewer hurdles around prescriptions, equipment usually available only in the hospital, and other medical assistance
At-home physical therapy visits
Coverage or respite care for caregivers

■ ■ ■ ■

PART IX
WHEN YOU'RE NOT
A STRAIGHT WHITE
MALE

■ ■ ■ ■

Because I'm a nurse, when I think about
the dignity of a country I think about its
healthcare system first, especially how it
takes care of its most vulnerable people.
Still, today, we have a great deal of work to
do. Systemic oppression, implicit bias, and
outright discrimination — realities now
more likely to be scrutinized across public
spheres — exist in the world of medicine.

Racism in healthcare is measurable. So

are sexism and cultural insensitivity. If the healthcare system is good at one thing, it's keeping a paper trail — meaning there's a record of every patient test result, intervention, and outcome, and those records can be analyzed across populations. When we want to see how we're doing in matters of health equity, the data is there to pull from — and it reveals that we are failing patients by many measures.

Research confirms that 40 percent of the time, black and Hispanic patients do not receive breast cancer treatment in line with guidelines.[1] All women experience misdiagnosis disproportionately to men.[2] Just under half of senior citizens have their pain dismissed by care providers as an expected part of aging.

"So which minority groups are you addressing in this book section?" my friend Maya asked over coffee last winter, and I started to rattle them off: *women, people of color, refugees, immigrants and asylees, people of lower socioeconomic status, transgender people, people with a history of trauma, sexual minorities, religious minorities, senior citizens, people with disabilities . . .*

I could have kept going, highly caffeinated and really on a tear at this point. She stopped me and asked the most intuitive, obvious question, which had slipped my mind while I was rambling: "When it has to do with being a patient, minorities are the majority, then?"

Yes. They are. We are. Many of us are minorities in some way, and most of us will at some point be vulnerable to discrimination in the care we receive. American healthcare, like many aspects of modern life, is most accessible and has the best outcomes for men who hold power. My intent is not to collapse all identities that are not straight, white, and male, nor to imply that the challenges they face in the healthcare system are the same. Rather, I hope to convey that care is constructed for — and most accessible to — the straight, young-to-middle-aged, abled, affluent white man.

Within the healthcare profession, there's a lot of talk and not enough action when it comes to these inequities. There are conferences and publications, but not enough mobilizing. And despite the prevalence of studies to the contrary, we too often think we're doing an okay job, that we, as a healthcare community, have transcended these malevolent practices, subconscious and otherwise.

My goal with this section is twofold.

First, I hope to inform you about the

modes of discrimination still functioning in modern medicine — to help you recognize them, name them, and mitigate their impact on the care you and those around you receive. Second, I hope to help you see healthcare as a lever to address social justice. Public health advocacy can only go so far until everyone (especially those with an advantage) understands the ways the system subjects their friends, neighbors, community members, and fellow citizens to inferior care. *If you can't trust a system to take care of those who are most vulnerable, you shouldn't trust it to take good care of you.* It's important for all of us to get curious, look around, and find ways to effect change.

TWENTY-FOUR: THE FEMALE PATIENT

Simone de Beauvoir once said: "Man is defined as a *human being* and a woman as a *female.*" Applied to medicine, this means there are patients, and then there are female patients.

From the earliest moments of its inception, medicine has been a story written for men. They are the subject of research, the template for intervention, and, often, the measure for advancement.

"Women's health" has been left up to men for the better part of history, and it's been annexed accordingly. Up until 1969, the phrase was synonymous with female reproductive function, reduced and confined to branches of procreation. In 1970, *Women and Their Bodies,* a course booklet that would a year later become *Our Bodies, Ourselves,* was published on stapled newsprint and sold for seventy-five cents. It was the first time women challenged the medical establishment en masse to improve health-care for women. Revolutionary in topic and tone, it drew attention to sex disparities in patient care and education that had been glossed over for decades.

The medical establishment didn't have much to say for itself, because data on women's health was scarce. It would be another twenty-three years before the National Institutes of Health Revitalization Act was passed, demanding that women and minorities be included in studies. It addressed the fact that beyond boobs and the uterus, medical research had largely disregarded half the population's unique medical needs for centuries.

Equitable medicine still isn't a reality. Women disproportionately endure adverse side effects, misdiagnosis, and flawed disease management. The lack of research specific to women also continues. Only a fraction of peer-reviewed medical journals require data to be analyzed by gender (note, such an analysis is more likely to occur if the principal scientist is a woman). There is a massive gap in dollars spent on research targeted to women as opposed to men, especially when it comes to leading conditions like heart disease and lung cancer. Women pay, on average, $90,000 more on healthcare over a lifetime than their male counterparts. The Food and Drug Administration (FDA) has, unsurprisingly, failed women too. Of all the drugs on the market that have been withdrawn for female-specific side effects, 80 percent were discovered after the drug was released.[1] At its worst, this patriarchal medical model is still used to control women in some parts of the country, especially when it comes to reproductive health, which can be seen in the way providers present care and treatment options.

But it's not just an equal-rights issue: Male and female bodies are not the same. Advancements in biological understanding consistently show that male and female bodies differ in ways that stretch far beyond hormones and reproductive systems. The differences are fundamental, extending across cells, organs, and the expression of diseases. For example: Hormones like estrogen impact cancer cell behavior. In heart disease, arterial plaques are dispersed differently in male and female blood vessels. Even the anatomy and physiology of our eyeballs are different, with diseases such as glaucoma and macular degeneration disproportionately affecting women.

First, let's discuss the issue of pain.

PAIN AND THE GENDER GAP

One major manifestation of the gender disparity in the practice of medicine is that mental and physical pain is considered and treated differently in women and men.

In a seminal 2001 study from the *Journal of Law, Medicine and Ethics,* "The Girl Who Cried Pain," authors found that while women have a higher prevalence of chronic pain syndromes and diseases associated with chronic pain than men, and women are biologically more sensitive to pain than men and respond differently to certain analgesics, women's pain reports are taken less seriously, and they receive less aggressive treatment for their pain. Women are more likely to have their pain reports discounted as "emotional" or "psychogenic" and therefore not real. They are less likely to receive pain medication when they report pain to their providers and are instead more likely to be given sedatives.[2]

How does this happen? Research indicates that medical providers are biased regarding the experience of female pain, leading them to discredit a woman's subjective report of pain until there is objective evidence and a scientifically ratified explanation for the pain's source. This bias, combined with 1) the cultural stereotype of women as hysterical creatures and 2) a medical world that often lacks sufficient understanding of female physiology, means that if you are a woman in pain, you're up against a lot.

What can patients do about it? First, just being aware that this phenomenon exists should empower you. Know that if you end up on the receiving end of it, it's probably not in your head. Trust your gut — and your experience of pain. Share the knowledge with your partners and friends, and if it comes down to it, cite the evidence to your provider in the moment. Point out that the data shows it's statistically likely that they are under the influence of a real and powerful bias that is affecting your care.

It's easier said than done, I know. But several passages in this book are meant to help you get comfortable standing up for yourself, calling out bias, being forthright when talking to providers, and using other sources of support to back you. In this case, pushing back against the system and advocating for yourself is imperative.

GENDER DIFFERENCES IN HEART ATTACKS

Another area where gender bias and inequitable research hits women particularly hard is heart attacks, the leading cause of death in the United States. Women and men have different hearts. They age differently, and the female reacts differently to stressors. In women, heart disease is more likely to develop in smaller branches of arteries. The plaque that leads to problems tends to be laid down more diffusely, making it more difficult to identify.[3]

Because of these differences and because of gender bias in understanding, treating, and preventing heart disease in women, women have worse clinical outcomes than men who suffer heart attacks. They're more likely than men to be incorrectly diagnosed and, if they survive the initial event, to die within twelve months.

Cardiologist Bernadine Healy, the first woman to head the National Institutes of Health (NIH), coined this phenomenon the Yentl syndrome. Like Yentl, the heroine of Isaac Bashevis Singer's nineteenth-century short story who was prohibited from studying the Talmud unless she dressed as a man, female patients are more likely to receive appropriate care for a heart attack if it presents like a male heart attack.

Because of this disparity, women need to take extra steps to ensure that the medical system handles their hearts carefully, having carte blanche to push back to ensure proper and thorough care in the event of a heart episode, which may indeed present differently than in their male counterparts.

Know the Symptoms

We associate heart attacks with an image of a ruddy man clutching his chest and dropping to the ground. But many women experience no such chest pain during a heart attack. Many have diffuse upper back, neck, and jaw pain, or a sensation that's more like squeezing pressure than pain.

Become familiar with the various and seemingly unconnected signs that a woman is having a heart attack. These include:

Shortness of breath
Unusual fatigue
Nausea
Lightheadedness or dizziness
Breaking out in a cold sweat
Pain in one or both arms
Unfamiliar pain in the upper body — back, shoulders, neck, jaw, upper abdomen
Squeezing motions racing up the spine
A feeling of indigestion when you haven't eaten in the last several hours
Chest pain or pressure, the feeling something is being wrung out, or the feeling

of an elephant standing on you

Trust the Signs

Society has conditioned women to downplay or dismiss their pain. Outsmart this pattern. If an odd, inexplicable sensation arises, trust it. Stop yourself from comparing it to what you *think* a heart attack looks like (in men), and consider the feeling against your own baseline. If you are at risk for heart disease and suddenly experience a novel and uncomfortable sensation of any sort, call 911.

Communication in the ER

When women have heart disease, their heart attacks are often misdiagnosed in ERs. To counter this, when relaying your story to the medical team in an acute situation, tell them that what you are experiencing is not your baseline. Explain your symptoms, be direct, and fight any tendency to downplay things. It's not a time to be stoic. A rule of thumb: In the ER, extreme pressure, even if it doesn't feel like pain, should be described as "chest pain." "Chest pain" is a code phrase that sets off a cascade of tests and investigations that women aren't afforded when symptom communication breaks down. Anyone experiencing what they think is a heart attack should not leave the ER without an EKG and a troponin test.

Follow-Up Care

Women also have to advocate for better follow-up care after suspected heart attacks. An angiogram is the gold standard for diagnosing a heart attack, but problems in the smaller arteries affected in heart disease in women are harder to identify with an angiogram. If symptoms continue even after a normal angiogram in the ER, follow up with a cardiologist.

REPRODUCTIVE AND SEXUAL HEALTH

One Key Question

I have a deep affinity for Oregon, where rain brings out character, and where even retainer walls along the I-5 are fecund with roses in the summer. It's also been considered a national leader in healthcare reform since the nineties, and it is the state with the best access to reproductive healthcare regardless of gender identity, insurance status, or citizenship.

Oregon has a history of setting itself apart, embracing innovation, and rejecting national guidelines to replace them with things that work better. One Key Question, a

477

project of the Oregon Foundation for Reproductive Health, is a striking example of this ingenuity. The initiative arose from a long-standing fragmentation of primary care and reproductive health services and is now transforming primary healthcare appointments for women and families around the country.

One Key Question addresses how healthcare providers support women in deciding if, when, and under what circumstances to get pregnant. It restructures primary care to support women in making reproductive health choices — whether they center on preventing pregnancy or having a healthy pregnancy — by ensuring that one simple question comes up at every routine appointment for women between the ages of eighteen and fifty:

Would you like to become pregnant in the next year?

If the answer is no, there's more to say than "great, keep taking birth control" (for women who have sex with men), because choosing birth control these days is like trying to pick out orange juice at the grocery store (some pulp, no pulp, from concentrate, organic, with mango . . .). There are short-term, long-acting, and reversible methods. Shots, pills, patches, implants, and intrauterine devices (IUDs). There are also new ways to access contraceptives — and various methods for reducing their out-of-pocket costs. The endless options make it important for providers to check in with women, revisit their options, and ensure they're satisfied with their current method.

If the answer to the One Key Question is yes, women can discuss conception with their primary care provider, which sets them up for a healthier pregnancy, even if it feels like a distant reality. Women are surrounded by information about avoiding pregnancy, but there's a dearth of information about how women can conceive in the healthiest way possible (whether they're trying to have a baby with someone of the opposite sex or the same sex, or on their own). And these conversations don't organically spring up at healthcare appointments.

Today, many women are older when they choose to become pregnant, meaning there's an increased likelihood they have a health condition or take medications regularly. And despite strong evidence and national initiatives to spread the word, only one in three women knows they need to take folic acid daily before conception to prevent major birth defects. Before conception, some women might want to get a screening for conditions that adversely affect pregnancy, or consider tweaking a prescription medication. Conversations with a provider before conception can answer important questions — including ones patients may not even know they should ask.

One Key Question illustrates a theme common to many sections in this book: It encourages making healthcare proactive instead of reactive, by initiating conversations in your PCP's office. If you're not in a state that's adopted this initiative, take One Key Question into your own hands. Before your appointment, ask yourself whether it's possible that you may want to become pregnant in the next year. Share the information with your provider using the following scripts:

"I do not want to become pregnant in the next year. I'm currently using _____ methods of birth control. Are there newer or alternative options that could be a better fit for me?"

Or:

"I'm considering becoming pregnant in

the next year. What can I do to ensure I'm as healthy as possible when I conceive?"

All people can bring up sexual and reproductive health issues related to pregancy during appointments. The initiative can and should take on a more gender-neutral approach. Our culture tends to place the responsibility for birth control, sexual health, and family planning on women, but, as my seventy-two-year-old dad said when proudly wearing his Planned Parenthood pin, "Until all women experience health security, it's everyone's problem!" In other words, you don't have to have a vagina to bring up these issues at appointments.

Addressing Pain and Fear around the IUD

The intrauterine device, or IUD, is a pretty miraculous form of birth control, but the anticipation of having one inserted is a significant source of anxiety for patients. On this matter, I linked up with the absolute best student from my nursing program, midwife Lucille Glick. She's not only a reliable, evidence-based encyclopedia of breast and vagina knowledge, but she also has a way of putting you at ease immediately. Here's what she had to say when I asked her what she'd tell both people who find the prospect of an IUD dread-inducing, and IUD veterans who would like to have a better experience during their next placement.

There is a spectrum of experiences with IUD insertion, from painful to hardly noticeable, with most people experiencing something in between. The sensation is often compared to strong menstrual cramps. The procedure is only a few minutes long, and discomfort is usually associated with three specific moments: when the tenaculum (an instrument used to position and stabilize the uterus) is placed, when the sound (an instrument used to measure the inside of the uterus) is inserted, and when the IUD itself is inserted.

Both physical and emotional factors can affect your IUD insertion experience: the position and shape of your uterus, your natural pain sensitivity, the provider's experience level, your relationship with your provider, any past history of sexual trauma, your level of comfort or anxiety regarding the procedure, your natural coping skills, and use of medications to reduce discomfort. Some of these factors are not modifiable, but many are.

There are a lot of things you can do to make sure your IUD insertion is as comfortable as possible. You will likely have an appointment with your provider before the IUD insertion to talk about what to expect. If you have never been pregnant, your provider might recommend scheduling your appointment during your period, when your cervix may naturally be more open, or they might prescribe a medication to help soften and open your cervix. They also might not! People who have never been pregnant can absolutely get IUDs, and many don't need to do anything for their cervix to be open enough.

A lot of clinics have a third person, sometimes called an escort, in the room during IUD insertions so the provider can focus on the procedure and someone else is available to focus on your comfort. If this isn't routine at your clinic, you can usually request it. You can also take an over-the-counter pain medication before your appointment. Make sure to take it far enough ahead of time that the medication will be effective during the procedure, and don't exceed the recommended dose.

There are also a lot of nonpharmacological things you can do to prepare. Brush up on relaxation skills, such as breathing techniques or visualization. Pick relaxing music to listen to in the waiting room, or even during the procedure. Talk with a calm and supportive friend. Better yet, bring your calm and supportive friend with you, or have them pick you up from your appointment. Plan something relaxing to look forward to afterward. But you don't have to do all of this, or even any of this, and your IUD insertion should still be fine.

The biggest takeaway is that concern about pain during the insertion process should not be a barrier to getting an IUD. If you think the IUD might be a good method for you but you're concerned about the insertion, talk with your provider. For patients more at risk of an uncomfortable insertion, such as people with anxiety, high pain sensitivity, or a history of sexual trauma, most providers are willing to prescribe anxiety or pain medication to help make the insertion process as comfortable as possible.

TWENTY-FIVE:
WHEN YOU'RE HAVING A BABY

Pregnancy brings many women and families into the world of medicine for the first time, an adventure that's dotted with great bouts of joy. Before we get there, though, let's discuss the more sobering realities about having a baby today.

More women die of pregnancy-related complications in the United States than in any other developed country. And only in the United States has the rate of death during labor and delivery been rising. Too many women die following childbirth every year in America, with women of color enduring the most extreme manifestations of this problem.[1]

The United States also has a higher infant mortality rate than any of the other twenty-seven comparably "wealthy countries," as defined by the Centers for Disease Control and Prevention. A baby born in America is more likely to die before their first birthday

485

than a baby born in Canada, Australia, Japan, or any developed country in Europe.

The issue of infant and maternal mortality in the United States is described in headlines as a "national embarrassment." It's also a public health crisis. How does this happen in a country where citizens spend more money on healthcare than in any other country in the world? A country where we're on the brink of creating an artificial pancreas and contact lenses that can detect blood glucose levels from tears? We are failing at one of the most primitive and fundamental practices in medicine for various reasons, among them that a large number of pregnant women go without access to prenatal and postpartum care.

As in other areas of medicine, race factors in as well. In a national study of the five major medical complications leading to maternal death and injury, black women were two to three times more likely to die than white women who had the same condition. And this problem can't be explained by educational level, or even accessibility of services. It persists despite the fact that the black midwife has served arguably the most vital role in advancing maternal health in the United States over the last centuries. It's accounted for by a grave pattern of the lives of black women being disrespected and dismissed by medical providers.

In January 2018, tennis dynamo and queen Serena Williams revealed she'd had a pulmonary embolism (a life-threatening event during which a blood clot breaks off and lodges in the lungs) following a cesarean section. She'd had one in the past, and she alerted her medical team to ask for an immediate CT scan and a blood thinner. The nurse attributed her request to confusion from pain medication, and the doctor did an ultrasound of her legs. She persisted and got the CT scan, confirming the embolism. Then she did a cover story for *Vogue* telling the public exactly what happened and calling attention to the problems inherent to modern labor and delivery systems.

For the majority of women, birth *is* a joy and a celebration, and their babies thrive. Furthermore, the deaths and severe complications associated with pregnancy are often preventable. Many nurse midwives and obstetricians are devoted to setting us on a new trajectory. My friends are among them. But to do it successfully will take active, and more refined, patient involvement.

In the labor and delivery ward, entering the world of medicine sight unseen at the final hour puts you at risk of a host of problems. Women and families can change the course of communication breakdowns between patients and providers, insufficient prenatal care, and inadequate teamwork. Having a strong relationship with your maternity care providers is paramount to a satisfying, safe childbirth experience. It may actually be the key determining factor, because a successful childbirth relies so much on planning and communication.

The following section provides guidelines and resources for navigating maternity care.

CHOOSING WHO, WHERE, AND HOW

Who

A number of different types of providers provide prenatal care, attend births, and care for women after birth in the United States. Most healthy women can choose from any of them. If you have a serious medical condition or are at high risk of developing a condition, plan to give birth in a hospital. Your primary care provider can give you more information on what situations might require specialized care.

Midwives

Midwives are generally thought of as emphasizing "mother-driven birth." Midwife deliveries are associated with:

Less use of pain medication, including epidurals, during labor[2]

Less use of episiotomy (a cut to widen the vaginal opening just before birth)[3]

Less use of forceps and vacuum during vaginal birth[4]

Increased initiation of breastfeeding[5]

Types of midwives include:

Certified nurse midwife
Certified professional midwife
Certified midwife

Certified nurse midwives have training in both nursing and midwifery — unlike other midwives, they are also registered nurse practitioners. They've graduated from a nurse-midwifery program accredited by the Accreditation Commission for Midwifery Education, they pass board exams like physicians do, and they are licensed by their state to practice nurse-midwifery. These are the majority of midwives, and in my opinion the best.

Physicians
The medical model of care is the one we think of when a woman has a baby in a

modern hospital with the help of a physician. This model of delivery is thought of as "doctor driven" as opposed to "mother driven," and there is generally more dependence on technology.

Providers include:
Ob-gyn physicians (obstetrician-
 gynecologists)
Some family practice physicians

Both models and both types of providers can be exceptional choices, depending on your needs, values, and medical condition. For further information on each, you can visit the International Childbirth Education Association (http://www.icea.org).

Where and How
Some women choose to give birth in hospitals, some at home, some in water, and some in outpatient centers. The specific policies, values, and practice methods of your birth setting can have a big impact on your care and outcome, so this is a major pregnancy decision.

When choosing where to give birth, consider that the setting and the provider are closely connected. When you are choosing a care provider, find out where that person attends births. Some physicians deliver babies outside the hospital, at birth centers; some midwives practice in hospitals. The American Association of Birth Centers (http://www.birthcenters.org) is an excellent resource for learning about the various settings in which one can give birth and exploring those in your vicinity.

The unexpected happens, and during a birth things can go wrong that require the presence of a physician trained in high-risk pregnancies, with access to technology and medication only available in full-fledged hospitals. For this reason, I lean toward recommending giving birth in a hospital. This is especially true if you have a high-risk condition. Make sure you are aware of the cascade of intervention (see later this chapter), and make a plan with your provider.

Insurance

As you make decisions about provider and birth setting, you will also want to make sure both accept your insurance. Call your insurance carrier directly and ask what specific services are and aren't covered, such as educational classes or working with a doula. Pregnancy is a qualifying event under the Affordable Care Act, so pregnant women can enroll in a healthcare plan at any time.

WAYS TO ADVOCATE FOR MOM AND BABY

Here is a nonexhaustive list of suggestions and recommendations for actions you can take during pregnancy, labor, and delivery to help them go as smoothly as possible:

Have checkups before and during pregnancy. Set a schedule for these early on with your primary care provider and ensure a smooth transition to your maternity care provider. The checkups will increase in frequency as the due date approaches.

Keep up with the dentist. The research is still new, but evidence points to the importance of good oral health for healthy birth outcomes. It can't hurt! Go to the dentist, just avoid X-rays.

If you have a mental health provider, loop them in. Women who take SSRIs (a type of antidepressant) may have to make decisions about going off them in order to breastfeed.

Find a doula. They're a pillar of support

during pregnancy and then labor and delivery, and they can help make sure you have the best experience possible.

If you don't like a provider, my advice is to switch. But if you're thinking of doing it during your last trimester, you'll have to carefully assess the risks and benefits of starting with a new person and developing a plan late in the game.

Before your delivery, ask your provider about the different options for managing pain, and create a plan together.

A WORD ABOUT INTERVENTIONS

The "cascade of intervention" principle means that one intervention during labor can set off others. Be informed about this in advance, so you can consider what matters to you and what contingency plans you may want in place. For example: IV pain medication may cause you to move around less during labor, necessitating the use of artificial oxytocin to speed up the labor, which could intensify contractions. This, in turn, could lead to an epidural, which ultimately slows things down and could necessitate a cesarean section. (C-sections and inductions can be essential, but they are also overused and come with risk. Talk to your provider to understand the specifics of each.)

The thing to remember with the cascade of intervention is that you always have the right to refuse a procedure, treatment, or course of action, and you can change your mind before and during labor.

IF YOU FEEL LIKE SOMETHING ISN'T RIGHT

The energy surrounding labor and delivery is frenetic. And birth is painful. Yes — even in the twenty-first century, *birth is painful!* Still, amidst the pain associated with a tiny human emerging from your body, there can be pain that doesn't feel normal, that isn't expected. It's easy for providers to dismiss a complaint of something being "off" as one of the normal pangs of childbirth. If you have a feeling something is off and you're told *that's normal,* do not let it go. Insist on a proper assessment. If you have a concern, ask that the provider stop what they are doing, get at your eye level, and listen.

AFTER DELIVERY

Ensure that a thorough examination is done every day you're in the hospital following childbirth to rule out infection in the vaginal tissue. Request that the handoff report (see the section "Bedside Report") is done at your bedside, in front of you and your family, during the change of shift.

TWENTY-SIX:
HEALTH ADVOCACY FOR
LGBTQ PATIENTS

The world is a different place now than it was in 1983, when San Francisco General Hospital created the first units in the world dedicated to those battling AIDS. It's a different place than it was in 1987, when homosexuality was listed as a mental disorder in the *Diagnostic and Statistical Manual of Mental Disorders,* and it's even a different place than in 2010, when same-sex spouses were kept from their partners in hospitals (see "You Define Family" for how to prevent this). Society has evolved, and it's past time the medical community caught up. Healthcare systems tend to cling to heteronormative and gendered frameworks, which comes at the expense of excluding patients.

Because of lacking competency in practice, women who have sex with women receive misleading information about their risk for cervical cancer or how often they should have Pap smears. Bisexual patients receive inconsistent and confounding information about STI transmission and contraceptive management. Transgender patients are forced to go out of their way for hormone therapy because their primary care clinic isn't up to date on basic practices, and on many intake forms they are excluded completely, having to chose between "male" and "female."

To sidestep this problem, it's key to have a provider with whom you feel comfortable. Talking about sex and gender up front can be a good litmus test for your overall rapport and fit. Next, the ideas below may help shape important conversations:

You do not need an explicit label for or definition of your sexuality when talking to a provider. You don't have to tell them the details of your sexual evolution.

Recommendations for Pap smear frequency are the same for all women, regardless of the sex of their partners. The test screens for cervical cancer, which can be passed through HPV — which all individuals can potentially carry.

Men who have sex with men should

discuss HIV and HPV screening with their provider. Have these discussions up front and tailor prevention.

STIs do not discriminate based on sexual orientation or gender identity. Risk comes down to the individuals engaging, their past history, and their health status, among other factors. Regardless of your sexual or gender identity, navigate safe sex and ask questions about your partner's status.

The LGBTQ population as a whole is at higher risk for certain chronic illnesses, likely because of historic marginalization of and prejudice against them in the healthcare system and society at large. These external, imposed stressors can impact mental and physical health. Your provider's office should be a safe space to discuss these issues. (If it's not, find a new provider.)

TRANSGENDER PATIENTS

My friend and research colleague Margo Presley is a Family Nurse Practitioner at the Multnomah County Health Department, in Portland, Oregon, where she works with some of the city's most underserved populations, including refugees and transgender youth. She's a model practitioner, incredibly thorough researcher, and an advocate for LGBTQ health. Below are some of her thoughts and recommendations for patients regarding this complex and often mishandled topic:

This one is a no-brainer, but don't go to any old PCP in your neighborhood if you are a sex or gender minority. Instead, go to a local LGBTQ resource and ask for recommendations, from agencies, friends, Facebook groups, etc.

If you can, talk to or e-mail with the provider or RN (someone from the clinic) before the appointment to try and find out about first appointments and what they entail so you can set your expectations accordingly.

If you have a support person you can bring to appointments (see page 112 on choosing an advocate), bring one! This can be a friend, family, or anyone you trust.

Providers are not objective beings without life experiences of privilege and oppression themselves. Chances are there is something that led them to do the work of serving LGBTQ patients, and it's perfectly okay to ask them how they got into it and what kind of ongoing training they seek out.

Co-set a flexible agenda with the provider. First visits are often about your past medical history, and if you have other goals for the visit make them known and try to negotiate what you can and can't accomplish in that visit. Remember, the saving grace of primary care is that it's incremental and ongoing. One can return as many times as it takes to address one's health goals.

Many health professionals are well-meaning but are steeped in the same heterosexist and cisgenderist culture everyone else exists in. Sadly, prepare yourself for being put into a category of cis or straight and how you might address that.

Questions about sexuality and gender identity should come up at the visit; it's basic information asked of everyone. The LGBTQ community has higher rates of

STIs so even though it's uncomfortable/ awkward for some, you *want* this to be brought up at your visit. It's a way for your provider to know you and know how to provide you with good care.

Know that you can refuse any exam. It may change the course of treatment, but if you're not comfortable with something, it's likely better to refuse it until you're ready rather than have a traumatizing experience and inauthentically consent to something. Even if you consent to an exam, you can stop it at any point. The provider should explain what they'll do and why before any exam.

You can agree on language to use for the body together, and ask providers to use that language throughout your time, just like they should use your correct name and pronoun.

Especially for trans patients, health maintenance and routine screening (cancer and otherwise) are important and occur less often. This may be in part because providers are less comfortable talking about one's anatomy and hormone history. A provider should be asking about what anatomy one has in a respectful way, couched in an explanation, so they know what to look for. Same with how long someone has been on hormone therapy, and if they went for prolonged periods without exposure to any hormones.

Regarding top surgeries, it's good to know if you have any breast tissue remaining (many people do for cosmetic reasons). Breast/chest cancer screening is still important, albeit done more commonly by ultrasound than mammogram.

The University of California, San Francisco (UCSF) has a great explanation on health maintenance and routine cancer and other screenings that are of extra importance for elder trans patients.

Regardless of sexual activity and sexual partners, the recommendation is to get a cervical cancer screening starting at age twenty-one and every three years until age thirty when one has "co-testing" of both cell changes (cytology) and HPV. If both are negative, it's every five years until age sixty-five, even if a cis woman has never had any kind of sex with a cis man.

TWENTY-SEVEN: IMPLICIT BIAS AND SYSTEMIC OPPRESSION

INSTITUTIONAL RACISM

In 1999, Congress asked the Institute of Medicine to answer the question: *Does quality of care differ based on a patient's race or ethnicity?* The answer was irrefutably affirmative — across every procedure, test, and diagnosis.

Medicine is far from the great equalizer. Race continues to impact healthcare delivery and grossly alter health outcomes. American Indians have a lower life expectancy than the US population at large by 5.5 years.[1] Latino/Hispanic populations have a 50 percent higher death rate from diabetes.[2] As discussed earlier, black women are three to four times more likely to die giving birth than white women.

The first source of institutional racism is racial variance in economic status, which impacts access to healthcare. Among full- and part-time workers in the United States, blacks in 2015 earned just 75 percent as much as whites in median hourly earnings. Hispanic men earned $12 for every $17 a white woman made. Among women across all races and ethnicities, hourly earnings trailed those of white men.[3]

The way money flows in and out of a household directly impacts access to health-care services. Yet despite the United States having one of the largest income-based health disparities in the world, racial differences in health outcomes *cannot* be explained solely by socioeconomic status. The problem extends beyond societal barriers to care, or the residential segregation that still exists in every major US city to cause them. Racism not only prevents individuals from accessing care, it's at play as they receive it.

If you're black or Hispanic, you're half as likely to receive pain medication in the ER for a broken bone than if you're white.[4] Black people are less likely to be admitted to the ICU than white people in critical situations. Black babies are 2.2 times more likely to die before their first birthday than white babies are. Out of the one million children diagnosed with appendicitis each year, 43 percent of white youth were prescribed opioids, relative to 21 percent of black youth.[5]

Something is happening to patients at appointments, in hospitals, and during procedures that indicates, in practice, care providers are devaluing the lives of non-white patients.

We've known this to be true for a long time. Research confirms repeatedly that medical racism is real and that the medical community's gestures to acknowledge it have in no way eradicated the problem.

In practice, racial discrimination takes several shapes. First, as *implicit bias.* As dangerous and insidious as outright discrimination, this kind of bias impacts teachers, cops, doctors, nurses, and civilians alike. Humans like to categorize. It's evolutionary, a mechanism of survival. From infancy, we use categories to assimilate information and navigate our surroundings. This means we're prone to stereotyping. If someone is "other" (or different from us) and we haven't had a dynamic variety of past encounters with this "other," we fall back on the most basic stereotypes society has provided to us.

In the case of medicine, this means minority patients can be treated as dangerous, promiscuous, drug-seeking, delusional, dishonest, more resistant to pain, less educated, and less capable of thriving.

The problem of implicit bias in medicine is compounded by non-factual belief systems still held by the medical community. In a 2016 study examining why black patients are systematically undertreated for pain relative to white patients, researchers found that half of white medical students and residents endorsed the idiotic belief that *black skin is thicker than white skin, and thus the population experiences pain less significantly.*[6] This egregious thinking, coupled with the considerable power these students and practitioners wield, is a disgrace.

Subconsciously or otherwise, these realities reflect a warped medical consciousness that has persisted in this country for decades. It's also a cycle that reinforces itself. Discrimination in clinical settings contributes to treatment nonadherence, influencing patient outcomes. It impairs communication between patients and providers, with patients rightfully discounting feedback and avoiding the healthcare system, exhibiting the stereotyped behavior and clinical outcomes which, in turn, reinforce provider beliefs and decision-making.

RESOURCES

Much of this book is prescriptive: what to know, what to do, where to turn when coming up against problems in the healthcare system that negatively impact your care. Because of the insidious nature of systemic racism, the answers on this topic are not straightforward. Those on the receiving end of medical racism are forced to make difficult decisions each time they seek out care. There's information about what to do if you're a provider and you encounter a racist patient, however there is a dearth of information about what to do when the roles are reversed, when the stakes and the costs are higher in every way. It's a vacancy that demands the medical community's sincere attention, and it's past time patients are included in the discussion on a mass scale.

The reality until then is, unjustly, that the onus is on patients to address racism as it unfolds before them. The tools and skills laid out in this book are intended to empower all patients in the face of adversity in the healthcare system. Below are additional resources that can inform you in these circumstances.

KNOW YOUR RIGHTS

Know your rights, and have a copy of them accessible to you whenever you enter a medical encounter.

As a patient, you have the right to:

Be informed about your care and options for treatment
Be treated considerately and respectfully
Be treated with privacy and confidentiality
Seek alternate opinions
Understand the legal reporting system
Know the cost of your care and options for paying for it
Leave your provider and seek treatment elsewhere

Per the Medical Code of Ethics, all patients have a right:

To courtesy, respect, dignity, and timely, responsive attention to his or her needs.

To receive information from their physicians and to have opportunity to discuss the benefits, risks, and costs of appropriate treatment alternatives, including the risks, benefits, and costs of forgoing treatment. Patients should be able to expect that their providers will provide guidance about what they consider the best course of action for the patient based on the provider's objective professional judgment.

To ask questions about their health status or recommended treatment when they do not fully understand what has been described and to have their questions answered.

To make decisions about the care the provider recommends and to have those decisions respected. A patient who has decision-making capacity may accept or refuse any recommended medical intervention.

To have the providers and other staff respect the patient's privacy and confidentiality.

To obtain copies or summaries of their medical records.

To obtain a second opinion.

To be advised of any conflicts of interest their provider may have in respect to their care.

To continuity of care. Patients should be able to expect that their provider will cooperate in coordinating medically indicated care with other healthcare professionals, and that the provider will not discontinue treating them when further treatment is medically indicated without giving them sufficient notice and reasonable assistance in making alternative arrangements for care.[7]

SEEK LEGAL REPRESENTATION

Law Help (https://www.lawhelp.org/resource/legal-aid-and-other-low-cost-legal-help) can help patients search for free legal aid programs by state and territory.

American Bar Association: Medical-Legal Partnerships Pro Bono Project, Washington, DC, Office 1050 Connecticut Ave. NW, Suite 400, Washington, DC 20036, 202-662-1000.

Disability Rights Legal Center (http://drlcenter.org/) is a nonprofit, public interest advocacy organization that champions the civil rights of people with disabilities as well as those affected by cancer and other serious illness. It includes the Cancer Legal Resource

Center (http://cancer legalresources
.org/).

MOBILIZE YOUR COMMUNITY

Community Catalyst (https://www
.communitycatalyst.org) is a place to
start. Its mission is to organize and
sustain a powerful consumer voice to
ensure that all individuals and communities can influence the local, state,
and national decisions that affect their
health.

Black Women's Health Imperative
(https://www.bwhi.org/) is a national
organization dedicated solely to improving the health and wellness of the nation's twenty-one million black women
and girls. It contains a number of resources on women's health.

The U.S. Department of Health and
Human Services Office of Minority
Health (https://minorityhealth.hhs.gov/
omh/content.aspx?ID=147&lvl=1&lvl
ID=3) provides information with a
primary focus on communities of color
within the United States and its ter-
ritories.

512

IF YOU DON'T SPEAK
THE LANGUAGE

Every patient has the legal right to a professional interpreter. To understand, ask questions, and engage in conversation about their health is a patient's fundamental right.

Providers can make the mistake of relaying health information in English to someone who doesn't speak it fluently. I've witnessed it in both community and hospital settings. Research has demonstrated that untrained people who serve as interpreters on an ad hoc basis (like family or friends of the patient, or someone who took the language in college) are more likely to make clinically significant mistakes than qualified medical interpreters. With all the medical jargon and legalese, it's often a challenge even for native English speakers to follow medical language in English.

It is a civil right to have access to an interpreter at a hospital, community clinic, or private practice. Clinicians are required by law to offer and facilitate this service up front. Medical interpreters are an essential part of the care team, and many hospitals have dedicated language service departments. When an interpreter is not available in person, there are phone-in services, as well as portable computerized devices that pull up a live interpreter.

Being denied an interpreter can result in longer hospital stays, greater risk of infections and falls, greater risk of readmission after being released, and ineffective management of chronic disease.

If English is not your first language, request that an interpreter is present at appointments and hospital stays, especially prior to surgery. If the situation is serious and no one delivers on this request, ask for a social worker.

If English is your first language and you witness someone else struggling to communicate in a medical setting, speak up.

IF YOU'RE A VET

Both my dad and my uncle served in Vietnam and were exposed to Agent Orange. They've had health problems as a result: my dad, diabetes, and his brother, Parkinson's. I've had a glimpse into the Veterans Affairs (VA) system, both through my family and through the older gents who regaled me with war stories during my days in geriatric care. I've met vets with MS, chronic heart failure, post-traumatic stress disorder (PTSD), and cancer — and what they say about the care they receive through the VA ranges from "piss-poor" to "exceptional."

Just like other hospitals, VA hospitals vary in quality, and some patients with serious health conditions even relocate to a region with a superior VA hospital. They can also seek out advocates well-versed in veterans' medical coverage. My dad didn't go out looking for an advocate when he was diagnosed years ago, but he got one, serendipitously, in the form of a secretary. When he was leaving one of his appointments, she looked at his paperwork and said, "Mr. Goldberg, you served in Vietnam in 1968, right? Well, it's likely this is Agent Orange, sir, and that means you qualify for disability. I want you to go to that desk right over there and ask them if you qualify."

Turns out — he did. He started receiving a check for $165 each month. A year later, it was bumped up to $1,500. This change was again due to luck — a friend of his who worked for the Veterans of Foreign Wars (VFW) told him that since he'd started taking medication for the disease, he qualified for 70 percent disability coverage instead of 10. Like all patients do, sometimes veterans will need to remind the VA system and its players how it is legally bound to help.

For veterans who have been diagnosed

with a new condition or are struggling with coverage or benefits, the VFW (http://www.vfw.org) is an excellent resource. It consists of a nationwide roster of volunteers who serve as professional advocates to help veterans cut through bureaucratic red tape. As my dad says, "They'll change the whisper of a veteran to the assertive roar of an advocate."

IF YOU HAVE A
SUBSTANCE-ABUSE HISTORY

If you've ever had a substance-abuse problem or you take methadone or Suboxone, it is important that you find care providers who will respect and communicate with you. Patients struggling with addiction today often find themselves in hostile environments during medical encounters, both at appointments and during hospital treatment. The result can be inadequate pain treatment or general care disparities due to defensive prescribing practices as discussed on page 264 ("Pain Management in an Opioid Epidemic").

If you fall into this category, this is a message to make sure that you and your primary care provider can communicate effectively. This will help you create plans for managing pain and addiction in tandem.

■ ■ ■ ■

PART X
WHEN YOU HAVE TO
STAND UP TO THE
INDUSTRY

■ ■ ■ ■

Twenty-Eight:
How to Deal with Insurance

At international healthcare conferences, arguing that a certain proposed policy would drive some country's system closer to the U.S. model usually is the kiss of death.

— Uwe Reinhardt

Insurance companies rarely feel like an ally. Most of us feel powerlessness and dread each time we're forced to pick up the phone and call one.

It may be this warped power distribution that leaves medical care without the privileges and rights implied and exercised in other consumer relations — despite the fact that we invest in it substantially over a lifetime. Insurance, private and public, is also an odd setup, as patients are a sideline to the economic exchange. A middleman pays your provider, so the bulk of the money doesn't come directly out of your pocket;

but the majority of us indeed pay — in deductibles and premiums, and the portions of income employers siphon off our paychecks. All the while, we cross our fingers that colossal bills won't show up in our mailbox unannounced.

Almost 90 percent of Germans receive coverage through a national public system, and these numbers are comparable in France and Canada. These countries have equitable systems with high access and quality, with the majority of healthcare coverage financed by the government, plus regulated competition in the private sector that drives quality and innovation without affecting patient spending. All in all, citizens can enjoy the ambient peace that comes with knowing that when something goes wrong, they will be taken care of.

Of course, that is not the case from where I write this book. The United States is a mixed bag — some private insurance is offered through employers, single-payer Medicare covers those over sixty-five, state-managed Medicaid is available to some, and semi-affordable coverage options exist through the Affordable Care Act Marketplace. And about twenty-eight million people are still uninsured.

The following sections break down various components of the insurance model to make it more approachable and easier to navigate. They include practices you can adopt on the front end to reduce costs, and they highlight ways to incorporate insurance checkpoints into your monthly routine so bills don't spring up on you.

INSURANCE 101

Most of the time, the frustrations that arise when calling insurance companies are rooted in communication issues. You may have found that the most difficult part of a phone call to your insurance is the act of explaining what you need help with. It's a tall order to sit on the line with a stranger and catch them up on the minute details or impossibly confusing predicament you find yourself in, and to tell them what you already know (so they don't repeat it) and what you need to know. And you may not even be sure what it actually is you need to know, when you don't speak insurance language.

Medical coding is how practitioners communicate with their billing staff, and how billing staff in turn communicate with insurance companies.

The process goes like this: A provider will walk into a room, discuss things with you, and maybe order various tests, conduct exams, or provide a medical treatment or intervention on the spot. The encounter is then transmuted into codes — procedural codes, diagnostic codes, medication codes. These codes are then transmitted to various parties to file away so they can settle up bills.

I won't bore you with a list of codes and how they're classified, but I will emphasize one thing: Whenever dealing with a medical bill of any sort, potential or otherwise, use the codes. Without them, trying to dispute a claim can induce a headache.

The codes are sort of like using a reference number for a customer service item or to pay a water bill — they ensure that you and the person on the receiving end are talking about the same thing. When you're setting off to determine a fair price for a procedure (see page 526), have the code for that procedure on hand. You can ask your provider during your appointment, or call the office later. When you're calling an insurance company to find out whether something is covered, use the code. If you've found a mistake on your medical bill, use the code to communicate with the call-center representative.

If you want to ensure that codes on your bill are accurate, you can look them up using the Physician Fee Schedule search feature on the Centers for Medicare and Medicaid Services website (http://cms.gov/apps/physician-fee-schedule/search/search-criteria.aspx).

Paying Up

Studies show that often the main culprit of avoiding care is that the patient does not understand basic insurance terms or provisions of the Affordable Care Act, and therefore does not understand what they are eligible for or what care will cost. Lack of basic health insurance literacy on this front causes people to miss preventive screenings or checkups, simply because they don't know that they're covered.

Here is a bare-bones, to-the-point explanation of the many things you pay the insurance company for and the expenses they share with you.

Deductible: The amount you must pay, out of your own funds, for healthcare services before your plan kicks in. This amount begins anew every year.

Premium: The amount you pay your insurance company every month to keep your plan active.

Co-pay: An established, flat fee you pay for appointments and prescriptions. It typically covers generic services like primary care appointments, specialist visits, and drugs. It kicks in once you've paid your deductible.

Coinsurance: The portion of expenses you are responsible for, outside of co-pays. For instance, if you have a hospital stay, your insurance might pay 80 percent and you would pay 20 percent, the coinsurance.

Maximum out-of-pocket: The maximum amount you could have to pay for healthcare services in a year. After you've paid this dollar amount, the coinsurance no longer applies and the insurance company pays 100 percent.

In-network: In-network providers are affiliated with the insurance network. Seeing them will cost you considerably less than seeing out-of-network providers.

WHAT PLAN IS BEST FOR ME?

The type of insurance plan that's best for you will vary based on where you are in life.

The decision (if you have a choice) should factor in your health status, income level, dependents, and options available to you based on your vocation. At a glance, all plans may seem exorbitantly expensive and tricky, so it's easy to divert your attention elsewhere and pick one without much consideration. The information outlined below can help you determine what you really need from a plan (beyond coverage in the event of an emergency) and how to get it in the most economical fashion.

Main Types of Insurance Plans

HMO: Health Maintenance Organization

Pros: Generally lowest costs and lowest premiums

Cons: Limited to in-network providers; need a referral to see a specialist

This plan is a good option for you if you are young and generally healthy, have a PCP in the plan's network, and need an economical plan.

PPO: Preferred Provider Organization

Pros: Large range of providers to choose from, and you can go out of network; do not need a referral to see a specialist

Cons: Generally higher costs

This plan is a good option for you if you need access to specialists, including if you have a chronic illness and want to be able to see specialists without a referral.

HDHP: High-Deductible Health Plan

Pros: Low premiums; plans typically arranged with employers; can deduct healthcare spending from taxes using a Health Savings Account.

Cons: Highest deductibles (at or above $3,000)

This plan is a good option for you if your employer offers it and you're in good health.

RADICAL WAYS TO SAVE MONEY

Healthcare Bluebook
Did you know a strep test for you or your child could cost $16, or closer to $80? That

MRIs and CT scans have some of the greatest price variations of all medical services, costing more at hospitals and less at freestanding clinics? That artificial insemination typically costs around $160 per treatment, but some clinics charge upward of $450 each time?

Just like for cars, there is a blue book for healthcare procedures, and it's a brilliant source of help when you're determining whether a fee for a test, procedure, or treatment is fair. It can save you tens of thousands of dollars with a few phone calls.

Prices are notoriously mysterious to patients. We know that a dress at Neiman Marcus costs tenfold what a dress at Target costs, and we anticipate higher prices on bread, milk, and dog food when we go to an organic market instead of a chain grocer. But we are not so privy to this price fluctuation in healthcare, and it can be astronomical (sometimes upwards of 500 percent). We're asked, *When do you want to do this? Monday or Thursday?* but never *How much do you want to pay for this?*

The rest of the story goes something like this:

Have the procedure. Get the bill. Panic.

Call the insurance company. See if there's been a mistake!

Instead, handle the money side of things up front with a few phone calls. It will take you approximately half an hour.

Every time your provider orders a test or schedules a procedure — from mole removal to endoscopy to brain surgery — follow these three steps. It's my hope that you adopt this protocol and become so familiar with it that it will be like cooking without needing a recipe.

Before you start, ask your provider for the specific name and CPT (current procedural terminology) code for what you're having and, most important, *where* they are sending you. (Literally the building, facility, or testing center.) If your provider is rushed, someone in the office can give you this information.

Step 1: Call the facility. Say the following:

"I'm scheduled to have a/an _____. The code is _____. My insurance plan is _____. I am calling to inquire what the cost will be."

If you are not using insurance, let them know you'll be paying up front and ask for a discount. (*Yes, like you're bartering at a flea market!*)

Step 2: Go to the Healthcare Bluebook, http://www.healthcarebluebook.com. Using this free resource, you can enter a test, hospital stay, surgery, exam, lab, medication, or imaging service, and then get a fair price quote based on your zip code. The results include a range and an explanation of the cost, even a breakdown of which portions go to the provider, the hospital, and other parties. You'll see that the facility, not the provider, is often the culprit of cost variation. Compare the quote against the price the facility gave you.

Step 3: If the quote from the facility satisfies you, you're good to go. If it doesn't, go back to your provider, explain the cost differential, and ask where else you can have the procedure done. They will have an alternative. If they're doing the procedure, often they will make their initial recommendation just based on which facility or hospital they are operating at on that day of the week.

Choose a different day and see where else they have privileges.

Comb Over Your Bills

In my household, receiving medical bills in the mail falls somewhere near running into a bitter ex on the things-to-dread scale. We are good at evading the situation until it's staring us in the face and we are staring back, as Joan Didion says, "with the nonplussed apprehension of someone who has come across a vampire and has no crucifix at hand."

Medical bills are rife with error. Studies indicate four out of five bills contain at least one.[1] It could be clerical, as minuscule as a misspelled patient name or an incorrectly entered digit — which could lead to an improper code, a denied claim, and a bill redirected to you. Procedures and tests can be inadvertently duplicated (meaning they are listed twice — and thus you are charged twice). Errors can come in the form of a mismatched diagnosis and treatment, as coded by the provider's office or the hospital. They can also occur when a provider's notes are sparse and the insurance company claims *insufficient medical necessity.*

Insurance coding is tricky, and each transfer through the call center to the billing department can make you feel more and more like you're playing a game of telephone. Who is looking out to make sure everything lines up? No one, if not you. The provider's job is only to submit the bill, and the insurance company has no problem passing it on to you if there's a mistake. Research estimates that billing errors amount to roughly $150 billion in overcharges annually — about $1,000 each year for a family of four.

Still, it's a tedious job to sleuth through a medical bill and look for errors. Below is an easy set of instructions for preventing and then fixing errors. Take a few minutes to do these each time you get a medical bill, *especially* if you weren't anticipating the amount.

Use page 521 to understand your insurance plan, at least at a basic level. You should have a general understanding of what charges to anticipate — such as copays and deductibles — so it's easier to catch things you shouldn't have been charged for.

Each time you have a medical encounter, be sure your name and date of birth are correct on the forms. Even an incorrect middle initial can lead to billing problems.

Look for duplicates, both within the bill in front of you and between that bill and one you have already received or paid.

Look for and save the Explanation of Benefits portion of the bill. You may need it when you're on the phone with the insurance company or the provider's office.

If you think there has been a mistake, call your insurance company and review the bill with them until you're satisfied with an answer.

Have independent medical billing experts review your bill. Use an online platform such as Simplee (http://www.simplee.com) or HealthCPA (http://www.healthcpa.com) to automatically search your bills for error. These services have apps through which you can upload snapshots of your bill.

A Quick Note About In- and Out-of-Network Providers

Even with planned, scheduled procedures, things may change in the final hour, causing an out-of-network provider to become involved without a patient's consent. This can result in four- or five-digit bills landing on unsuspecting patients. Many states are passing laws to prohibit these "surprise" costs.

Providers should be either in network or out of network, but it's not always that simple. Some can be in network for certain procedures but not others. Always check with the provider up front about whether any service they provide is *not* covered, or go straight to the source and ask your insurance carrier.

Over-the-Counter Savvy

Over-the-counter savvy is not directly related to insurance, but it is related to economics. Possessing it can save you enough money over the years to take a trip to Aruba.

As you've likely picked up on by now, capitalism rules the healthcare industry just as it does other aspects of our lives. From sea to shining sea, from capsule to cream to pill. We see as many advertisements for Tylenol as we do for Subarus, Tide, and Snickers.

Even when it comes to medications, marketing is always at play. Brand names carry nostalgia, which translates to comfort, and what more do you want when you're sick? When I was a baby, it was Vicks Vapo-Rub and a nap on the sheepskin rug. When I was in school, it was packets of Luden's cherry throat drops tucked in my desk. To this day, I'm convinced those products are the ticket.

It's hard to transcend the power of branding, but when it comes to over-the-counter medications — be a cool customer and buy generic. Each and every drug has a trade or brand name and a generic name. Tylenol is the trade name for acetaminophen and Claritin is the trade name for loratadine, for example. You can check page 153 for a list of common brand names and their generic counterparts, but you can usually also turn a package or bottle around, look at the label, and find the active ingredients. The active ingredients in the generic, less-expensive version of a medication are usually identical to those in the brand-name version.

We can thank Benjamin Franklin, who paved the way for the United States Pharmacopeia (USP). The USP verifies a drug's identity, potency, purity, and performance. All drugs sold on the US market must meet its standards.

Unlike for drugs, though, compliance with

USP standards is optional for vitamins, minerals, and supplements, so it's important to look for the USP stamp on them. For example, these products are not required to conduct clinical trials prior to market entry. Do your research to find the best brands. If you're not sure where to start, Labdoor (http://www.labdoor.com) is an excellent, well-designed resource for determining how to best spend your money on dietary supplements — from creatine to fish oil — whether they are recommended by your doctor or taken by personal choice.

Last, if your primary care provider recommends a particular dietary supplement or if there's one you go through regularly, ask for a prescription. Going this route can be significantly less expensive, even without insurance.

GETTING CARE WHEN YOU'RE UNINSURED

People without insurance used to be able to use emergency rooms as their de facto PCP whenever a health issue arose. ERs cannot turn anyone away and must provide care regardless of the patient's ability to pay. Today, though, it's not so simple. If you're uninsured, you can still go to the ER, of course, but you may be crushed with a bill a few weeks later. This is why when you're admitted, someone always collects your contact information. It's a friendly version of *we know where you live.*

If uninsured, once you arrive, *never* let a hospital reroute you to another facility because you can't pay. Demand that you're treated where you are, and if you're met with resistance give everyone a gentle reminder of the law — because sending you elsewhere and delaying your treatment is not only unethical but also illegal.

If you're uninsured or between coverage and need general care, you may be inclined to wait it out until your situation changes. But there are resources available to you that can help, and the sum of their parts is almost as solid as an insurance plan when it comes to preventive care.

Private-practice clinics: More often than not, a primary care provider will see you even if you don't have insurance. The caveat (and it's Mafia-esque, I know) is that you have to pay in cash up front. Call clinics near you and ask if this is an option, and what discounts they offer if you pay this way. Most will offer a discounted rate, and you can get that in writing before services are rendered.

Urgent care: For a detailed explanation of when and how to use urgent care, see the section "Choose Urgent Care If . . ." Urgent care centers accept payment without insurance, and their fees and wait times are much less harsh than those of emergency rooms.

Walk-in clinics, community clinics, nonprofit clinics: Larger hospitals often have satellite clinics in medically underserved communities and in large urban settings. Services at such clinics are typically low-cost or done on a sliding-scale basis. Find Care (http://www.findcare.org) produces a list of all free and low-cost clinics in your vicinity based on your zip code.

Hospital events: In most cities, major hospitals and medical centers consistently engage with their communities via open-to-the-public events. Most boast multiple flu-shot clinics during fall months, provide free cholesterol and blood pressure readings, and offer all kinds of health screenings to catch and prevent diseases from breast cancer to melanoma. Sign up for newsletters from the major hospitals in your area, and you will get updates about all the free clinics and screenings you can take advantage of as a community member.

If paying for medications is a hardship or a barrier to care, patient assistance programs may help. Many state and corporate prescription assistance programs help patients obtain free or nearly free medicines if they qualify. Apply online at http://www.pparx .org.

Unfortunately, and not by coincidence, some of these programs make the application confusing and difficult to fill out, which deters most people. But community centers, churches, and charity organizations may offer resources to help you fill them out. Call them up and ask if they have people or groups that can help you fill out an application.

Another way to save money on medications is to ask your provider if you can get a higher dose and cut the pill in half. This often saves patients substantial money out of pocket.

Twenty-Nine:
Big Pharma and the FDA

Drug Reps and Olive Garden: Conflicts of Interest

Among my memories of being a kid are our doctor mom taking us along for "drug-rep dinners." Sometimes they were at Olive Garden, sometimes at fancier places that served steak on carts. These were rare occasions, my brother and I allowed to choose anything on the menu we liked and my parents getting a bottle of nice wine that put them in a grand mood.

Sometimes these same drug reps who chatted people up at the dinner parties would show up at my mom's office when I was in tow. They would waltz in, rolling suitcases with blister packs of samples and trays of turkey-and-cream-cheese sandwiches. They'd smile and hand me a branded pen I'd feel special using at school. *Wow, they're so nice!* I'd think. It was the early nineties, and it was all very jovial.

Today it's unlikely there would be such soirees at the Olive Garden, with wining and dining funded by Big Pharma.

Over half of today's providers have put the kibosh on these visits and closed their doors to drug reps. According to a study published in *JAMA Internal Medicine,* a single meal with a drug rep is all it takes to make a physician more likely to prescribe an expensive brand-name statin instead of a less expensive generic statin.[1] Other studies have found that older, generic versions of drugs perform as well as or better than the modern, expensive equivalents prescribed in their place — so these drug-rep dinners make clinical effectiveness and price considerations go out the door.

New laws and practices today ensure that relationships between prescribers and drug reps are kosher. Drug reps now have to report every exchange of value worth ten dollars or more between their companies and prescribers to the Centers for Medicare and Medicaid Services, making it difficult for them to get away with the seedy exchanges of times gone by.

Yet like all dark arts, such influence still makes its way into government and medicine, including the decisions your providers make in choosing medications to prescribe.

And it doesn't stop at medications: This under-the-table handshake can extend to medical equipment, research (as we'll talk about next), and even the rods, screws, and prosthetics surgeons use to fix a broken hip.

The FDA has its own set of influencers. Here, a drug goes through a preclinical phase and then three clinical phases, which can start with as few as ten patients but reach up to three thousand by phase three. Between the various phases, the drug must consistently demonstrate its efficacy, safety, and superiority to alternatives on the market. After that, an application for sale on the market is submitted to an FDA advisory committee — a process that takes months to years.

This process sounds solid, but it's heavily influenced by money changing hands. More than half of the funding for the FDA's Center for Drug Evaluation and Research comes from drug companies. An already flawed FDA is in further jeopardy today, as the current US administration aims to down-regulate and lower evidentiary standards, advocating for drugs to be approved before they are shown to work and letting people take them at their own risk.

When I'm the patient, I'm generally wary of any prescription for a fancy new medication when there are generic equivalents shown to do perfectly well. It usually merits a little digging. So if you are prescribed an expensive brand-name medication, question further, especially if you're paying out of pocket. When a provider wants you to buy a specific brand of equipment, ask if there's a less expensive alternative. The drug nomenclature resource on page 153 can help you find generic equivalents, which you can then ask your provider and pharmacist about (see page 108 for soliciting help from a pharmacist).

WHAT DOES "EVIDENCE-BASED" REALLY MEAN?

Evidence-based. It sounds smart, secure, a welcome qualifier in a landscape of confusing, often conflicting information. It's the backbone of change and progress in the medical community, and we lean into it accordingly.

But change is the only constant. The issue with evidence-based practice and the validity we assign to it in healthcare is that evidence often evolves faster than the human systems that apply it. It has a shelf life, determined by whatever research is about to replace or discredit it. It often becomes antiquated just as it's put to use. On the other hand, medicine can be quick to adopt new practices based on flimsy evidence. There's a range of quality and efficacy even in evidence-based practice.

There are also boulders in the stream — old, stale, less glamorous practices that hold their ground like burned-out professors with tenure: It's distressingly common for patients to receive treatments that the evidence has established are ineffective. For example, each year close to a million Americans receive a stent placement to open up a blocked artery. A stent can be lifesaving, but it's well established that the procedure is overdone and frequently unnecessary; almost half the time, it poses no benefit and considerable risk to the recipient.[2] Stent placements are a boulder — around which an entire industry has been built. The survival of that industry depends on the procedure maintaining its status as the go-to solution for coronary artery disease.

Why are we exposed to surgical interventions that pose no benefit? Because there is no regulation of surgical procedures — not by the FDA or by any equivalent administrative board.[3]

Now that you're informed, every time your provider recommends a procedure, ask more questions and engage them in an open dialogue about the procedure's nature and history.

EVIDENCE-BASED OR MARKETING-BASED?

If you recall the Premarin and Prempro scandal from the early 2000s, you might remember that Wyeth pharmaceutical company, owned by Pfizer, had to pay close to $700 million in lawsuits because nearly ten thousand postmenopausal women reported getting cancer after taking the artificial hormones Premarin and Prempro. Subsequent litigation revealed that between 1998 and 2005, the company had paid ghostwriters to fabricate scientific papers — twenty-six in total, published in eighteen medical journals including the *American Journal of Obstetrics and Gynecology* — promoting the safety and efficacy of the drugs and downplaying or omitting data on their side effects, and then found and paid physicians to sign them and get them into major scientific journals.

It's a classic case reminding us that how we (and our providers) assess medical research might be very different if we understood the study's origins.

When it comes to authenticity in research and practice, there is a source of hope in the next generation of practitioners. In recent years, the American Medical Student Association (AMSA) implemented an initiative called Just Medicine. Developed by a group of medical students around the country, their slogan is: *No Kickbacks. No Speakers Bureaus. No Free Samples.* Among their accomplishments: They've created a scorecard to grade academic medical centers "on the presence or absence of a policy regulating the interactions between their students and faculty and the pharmaceutical and device industries." You can check out the list at http://www.amsascorecard .org. It's not exhaustive, but you might find the major medical center in your city. In 2008, AMSA partnered with the Pew Prescription Project, an initiative of the Pew Charitable Trusts, to develop rigorous and transparent methodology to assess the policies at medical schools throughout the country.

When it comes to keeping costs down for medications, use the resources in this book to ask questions about price and alternative generic options whenever you're prescribed a medication. Next, remain politically engaged, and support candidates working to bring down pharmaceutical costs. Always be informed, and do extra legwork on your own to vet the studies on which your provider's recommendations are based.

Final Words

With this, I wish you happiness and confidence as you move forward in navigating the world of modern medicine.

Go in good health.

546

ACKNOWLEDGMENTS

Thanks are in order to those who believed in this idea at critical moments and set it on the path to becoming a book. To the infallible Allison Hunter and Clare Mao. To Sarah Murphy, who began as my editor and ended up my friend. To editor Hannah Robinson for gracefully shepherding me along. To Seb King, Lisa Tumarkin, Helen Haskell, Margot Presley, Lucille Glick, and Adrian Murphy for their essential input. To Julie Hersh for her sharp eyes, narrator Anne Marie Gideon, and the Harper Wave family at large.

Next, cheers to solid gold friends, without whom this book would have been written with half the heart. To Mamie Stevenson, who got me writing. To Maddy Villano, who appears around the corner at all the right moments. To Gabe Zinn, who took me to the Lucky Horse Shoe, and to the Malek-

Axleys, who took me in the summer I started this project. To Jillian Porten's charm, Nick Hiebert's exuberance, and Stephanie Cantor's advice. To muse Clemmie Wotherspoon and mentor Maya West. To Lilly and Peter Nickerson for the fishing and cormorants. To Kayla Wisnieski, Carolyn Griesser, and Jazmyn Price for welcoming me to a new city, and to Margaux Forsch, Garrett Felber, and baby Jules for visiting me there.

Thanks to my mom, who introduced me to the world of medicine, and to my dad for being my steadfast friend. To my grandparents Dorothy and Sidney, and my brother Ethan. I am lucky to call my family my friends, and to those touched this book directly — either by listening to me as I talked out an idea or sharing their own story — I am especially grateful: Julie Kaplan, Amy Sgro, Sarah Sgro, Molly Kaplan, Phyllis Mossberg, Deborah Goldberg, and Elizabeth Kelley.

To patients. To teachers (Pete Rock, Kristen Beiers-Jones, and Paul Currie). And to libraries.

To Bourbon the dog.

And, of course, to Tess.

We ate and talked and went to bed,
And slept. It was a miracle.

APPENDICES

PEDIATRIC VACCINATION SCHEDULE

VACCINATION SCHEDULE (CDC)	
Birth	Newborn blood screen Hepatitis B (Hep B)
3–5 days	Well-child visit
7–14 days	Well-child visit
2 months	Well-child visit DTaP (diphtheria, tetanus, acellular pertussis) Hep B Hib (Haemophilus influenzae type B) IPV (polio) PCV (pneumococcal vaccine) Rotavirus (given by mouth)
4 months	Well-child visit DTaP Hib IPV PCV Rotavirus (given by mouth)

VACCINATION SCHEDULE (CDC)	
6 months	Well-child visit DTaP Hep B Hib (if needed) IPV PCV Rotavirus (given by mouth)
9 months	Well-child visit
12 months	Well-child visit Hepatitis A (hep A)—not before first birthday Hib MMR (measles, mumps, rubella)—not before first birthday PCV Varicella (chicken pox)—not before first birthday
15–18 months	Well-child visit DTaP Hep A Any twelve-month immunizations not already given
2 years	Well-child visit
3 years	Well-child visit
4 years	Well-child visit DTaP IPV MMR Varicella

VACCINATION SCHEDULE (CDC)	
5 years	Well-child visit
6, 8, and 10 years	Well-child visit
11 years	Well-child visit HPV (human papillomavirus)—two doses, with six months between first and second dose MCV (meningococcal vaccine) Tdap booster (tetanus, diphtheria, acellular pertussis)
12 years	Well-child visit
13 years	Well-child visit Varicella blood test, if vaccine not given and no history of chicken pox
14 and 15 years	Well-child visit
16 years	Well-child visit MCV booster
17 years	Well-child visit

ROUTINE EXAM SCHEDULE

You should get routine preventive care exams at the following times:

ROUTINE EXAM SCHEDULE	
Birth	
1 week	Well-child Exams
2 weeks	Well-child Exams
1 month	Well-child Exams
2 months	Well-child Exams
4 months	Well-child Exams
6 months	Well-child Exams
9 months	Well-child Exams
12 months	Well-child Exams
15 months	Well-child Exams
18 months	Well-child Exams
2 years	Well-child Exams
2.5 years	Well-child Exams
3 years	Well-child Exams
Age 5–18	Annually
Age 18–21	Annually
Age 21–49	Every 1–3 years depending on need/risk factors (talk with your PCP to determine how often you should plan them)
Age 50+	Annually

WHAT TYPE OF PATIENT AM I?

I grumble about "type" quizzes and tend to shun them. They're reductive — no one fits perfectly in a box. Still, people as patients often cling to a few specific tendencies out of a combination of personality, health history, and adaptive mechanisms. Consider the types below and see if you recognize yourself, or at least the ways these different traits might manifest in you. Don't think of it as an assessment of your whole being, but rather of how you respond to medical stimuli.

The Laissez-Faire
Patients of this type keep cool and don't bother themselves with the details, usually deferring to the experts. They may nod whether or not they fully understand a provider's instructions, and they trust that all medical intervention is warranted.

The challenge: to stay curious and aware,

and assert agency.

The Health-Anxious

Patients of this type tend to err on the side of caution and never stray far from the locus of control when it comes to their health. These patients are likely to reference a message board at their appointment, or put themselves through extensive testing "just in case." When their energy is channeled properly, they might catch something the system misses, but they're prone to more confusion and conflict with providers along the way.

The challenge: to be confident and informed, rather than make decisions based on fear.

The Professional

My mother, an ob-gyn, used to chase me around the kitchen with a flu shot and scoff at a low-grade fever, so I know this type well. Then I became one! (Fortunately, thanks to my dad's side of the family, I've got a good dose of hypochondria to keep it balanced.) Healthcare professionals can go different ways when it comes to their own healthcare. Some lean too far into the DIY approach. Knowing too much is both a superpower and a weakness.

The challenge: to turn to professional help when it's warranted.

The Avoidant
Patients of this type might like to remind everyone that their grandfather happily avoided the doc through his nineties and was none the worse. They might tend to let things go, avoiding visits and screenings at all costs, dealing with things at the final hour.

The challenge: to face the music — because none of us gets out of this life without a medical hiccup or two.

The Private Stoic
Either it's not their first rodeo, or they have excellent meditation skills. Patients of this type typically have high pain thresholds and appear outwardly calm and collected despite discomfort. They also tend to be private in matters concerning health. It takes more than the average crisis for them to approach the healthcare system.

The challenge: to effectively convey their experiences so others can help.

Some people might need to open up more, some less. Some need extra structure to stay on top of their healthcare, whether to catch a disease before it's life-threatening or to make sure their vaccinations are up to date. Some need a little push to remember that the system is flawed and they shouldn't trust in it blindly. Being aware of your own tendencies can guide you in choosing the best people to get on your medical team, and communicating effectively with them.

COMMON HOSPITAL STAFF

Nursing
  Chief nursing officer (CNO)
  Director of nursing services
  House supervisor
  Nurse manager
  Charge nurse
  Staff nurse
  Certified nursing assistant (CNA)

Medicine
  Medical director
  Head of department
  Attending physician or hospitalist
  Fellow
  Chief resident
  Senior (usually third-year) resident
  Junior (second-year) resident
  Intern (first-year resident)
  Medical student

Other Professionals
Pharmacist
Registered dietician
Respiratory therapist
Speech therapists
Occupational therapists
Physical therapists
Child life specialist
Social workers
Case managers
Chaplains

Whenever somebody walks into your hospital room, ask them to identify themselves.

MEDICAL JARGON[1]

a.c.: Before meals (when to take a medication)

ACL: Anterior cruciate ligament of the knee

Ad lib: At liberty; at the patient's leisure

ADH: Antidiuretic hormone

ADHD: Attention deficit hyperactivity disorder

ADR: Adverse drug reaction

ANED: Alive, no evidence of disease

Anuric: Not producing urine

ARDS: Acute respiratory distress syndrome

ARF: Acute renal (kidney) failure

ASCVD: Atherosclerotic cardiovascular disease

b.i.d.: twice daily (how often to take a medication)

BMP: Basic metabolic panel

BP: Blood pressure

BPD: Borderline personality disorder

Ca: Cancer; carcinoma

CABG: Coronary artery bypass graft

C&S: Culture and sensitivity (to detect infection in a wound or the throat)

cap: Capsule

CBC: Complete blood count

CC: Chief complaint

cc: Cubic centimeters

Chem panel: Chemistry panel indicating the status of the kidneys, liver, and electrolytes

C/O: Complaint of (the patient)

COPD: Chronic obstructive pulmonary disease

CPAP: Continuous positive airway pressure (a machine)

CT: Chemotherapy

CVA: Cerebrovascular accident (stroke)

D/C or DC: Discontinue or discharge

DCIS: Ductal carcinoma in situ (a type of breast cancer)

DDX: Differential diagnosis (indicates that several diagnostic possibilities are actively being considered)

DJD: Degenerative joint disease (another term for osteoarthritis)

DM: Diabetes mellitus

DNR: Do not resuscitate

DOE: Dyspnea on exertion (shortness of breath while active)

DTR: Deep tendon reflexes (when tested with a rubber hammer)

DVT: Deep venous thrombosis (blood clot in large vein)

ETOH: Alcohol (in history or intake)

FX: Fracture

g: Gram

gtt: Drops (eye, ear, etc.)

HA: Headache

H&H: Hemoglobin and hematocrit (used to assess anemia)

H&P: History and physical examination

H/O or h/o: History of

HRT: Hormone replacement, or hormone replacement therapy

h.s.: at bedtime (when to take a medication)

HTN: Hypertension

I&D: Incision and drainage

IBD: Inflammatory bowel disease

ICU: Intensive care unit

IMP: Impression (of the provider or therapist)

in vitro: In the laboratory

in vivo: In the body

JT: Joint

K: Potassium

KCl: Potassium chloride

LBP: Lower back pain

LCIS: Lobular carcinoma in situ (a type of breast cancer)

LLQ: Left lower quadrant of the abdomen

LUQ: Left upper quadrant of the abdomen

Lytes: Electrolytes (potassium, sodium, carbon dioxide, and chloride)

mg: Milligrams

M/H: Medical history

ml: Milliliters

npo: Nothing by mouth (fasting before surgery or while recovering)

NSR: Normal sinus rhythm (of the heart)

N/V: Nausea or vomiting

O&P: Ova and parasites (stool O&P is tested in cases of chronic diarrhea)

O.D.: Right eye

O.S.: Left eye

O.U.: Both eyes

p: After meals (when to take a medication)

PERRLA: Pupils equal, round, and reactive to light and accommodation (a term used during routine exams)

PFT: Pulmonary function test

p.o.: By mouth (how to take a medication)

PRN: As needed (a medication or intervention)

PT: Physical therapy

PTH: Parathyroid hormone

PTSD: Post-traumatic stress disorder

PUD: Peptic ulcer disease

"Q": (From the Latin *quaque*) indicates how often to take a medication

q2h: Every two hours

q3h: Every three hours

qAM: Each morning

q.d.: Each day

qhs: At bedtime

q.i.d.: Four times daily

qod: Every other day

qPM: Each evening

RA: Rheumatoid arthritis (joint disease)

RLQ: Right lower quadrant of the abdomen

R/O: Rule out (diagnosis)

ROS: Review of systems (indicates the provider has reviewed all organ systems, from skin to neurological function to liver)

RUQ: Right upper quadrant of the abdomen

SOB: shortness of breath

SQ: Subcutaneous (an injection that goes just under the fat layer of the skin)

T: Temperature (recorded as part of the physical examination — it is one of the "vital signs")

TAH: Total abdominal hysterectomy (surgery to remove a woman's reproductive organs)

THR: Total hip replacement

t.i.d.: Taken three times daily (a medication)

TKR: Total knee replacement

TMJ: Temporomandibular joint and associated issues

UA or u/a: Urinalysis (common upon admission to hospital)

ULN: Upper limits of normal

URI: Upper respiratory infection (cold or sinusitis)

UTI: Urinary tract infection

VS: Vital signs (temperature, blood pressure, and pulse)

Wt: Weight (body weight, usually recorded in kilograms)

XRT: Radiation therapy

FREE SCREENINGS AND SERVICES*

Services for All Adults

Abdominal aortic aneurysm one-time screening for men of specified ages who have ever smoked

Alcohol misuse screening and counseling

Blood pressure screening

Cholesterol screening

Colorectal cancer screening for adults over 50

Depression screening

Diabetes (type 2) screening

Diet counseling

Hepatitis B screening for people at high risk

Hepatitis C screening for adults at increased risk, and once for everyone born between 1945 and 1965

* Covered by all Marketplace insurance plans and most other major insurance plans.

HIV screening for everyone ages 15 to 65, and people of other ages at increased risk

Immunization vaccines (see page 554)

Lung cancer screening for adults ages 55 to 80 who have smoked

Obesity screening and counseling

Sexually transmitted infection (STI) prevention counseling

Syphilis screening

Tobacco use screening for all adults, and cessation interventions for tobacco users

Other Covered Preventive Services for Women

Breast cancer chemoprevention counseling for women at higher risk

Breast cancer genetic test counseling (BRCA) for women at higher risk

Breast cancer mammography screenings every one to two years for women over 40

Cervical cancer screening for sexually active women

Chlamydia infection screening for younger women and other women at higher risk

Domestic and interpersonal violence

screening and counseling for all women

Gonorrhea screening for all women at higher risk

HIV screening and counseling for sexually active women

Human papillomavirus (HPV) DNA test every three years for women with normal cytology results who are 30 or older

Osteoporosis screening for women over age 60, depending on risk factors

Rh incompatibility screening follow-up testing for women at higher risk

Sexually transmitted infections counseling for sexually active women

Syphilis screening for women at increased risk

Tobacco use screening and interventions

Well-woman visits to get recommended services for women under 65

Services for Pregnant Women or Women Who May Become Pregnant

Anemia screening on a routine basis

Breastfeeding comprehensive support and counseling from trained providers, and access to breastfeeding supplies, for pregnant and nursing women

Contraception: Food and Drug Administration–approved contraceptive methods, sterilization procedures, and patient education and counseling, as prescribed by a healthcare provider for women with reproductive capacity (not including abortifacient drugs). This does not apply to health plans sponsored by certain exempt "religious employers."

Folic acid supplements for women who may become pregnant

Gestational diabetes screening for women 24 to 28 weeks pregnant and those at high risk of developing gestational diabetes

Gonorrhea screening for all women at higher risk

Hepatitis B screening for pregnant women at their first prenatal visit

Rh incompatibility screening for all pregnant women and follow-up testing for women at higher risk

Syphilis screening

Tobacco intervention and counseling for pregnant tobacco users

Urinary tract or other infection screening

Services for Children

Alcohol and drug use assessments for adolescents

Autism screening for children at 18 and 24 months

Behavioral assessments for children ages: 0 to 11 months, 1 to 4 years, 5 to 10 years, 11 to 14 years, 15 to 17 years

Blood pressure screening for children ages: 0 to 11 months, 1 to 4 years, 5 to 10 years, 11 to 14 years, 15 to 17 years

Cervical dysplasia screening for sexually active females

Depression screening for adolescents

Developmental screening for children under age 3

Dyslipidemia screening for children at higher risk of lipid disorders ages: 1 to 4 years, 5 to 10 years, 11 to 14 years, 15 to 17 years

Fluoride chemoprevention supplements for children without fluoride in their water source

Gonorrhea preventive medication for the eyes of all newborns

Hearing screening for all newborns

Height, weight, and body mass index (BMI) measurements for children ages: 0 to 11 months, 1 to 4 years, 5 to 10 years, 11 to 14 years, 15 to 17 years

Hematocrit or hemoglobin screening for all children

Hemoglobinopathies or sickle cell screening for newborns

Hepatitis B screening for adolescents at high risk

HIV screening for adolescents at higher risk

Hypothyroidism screening for newborns

Immunization vaccines for children from birth to age 18 (see page 551)

Iron supplements for children ages 6 to 12 months at risk for anemia

Lead screening for children at risk of exposure

Medical history for all children throughout development ages: 0 to 11 months, 1 to 4 years, 5 to 10 years, 11 to 14 years, 15 to 17 years

Obesity screening and counseling

Oral health risk assessment for children ages: 0 to 11 months, 1 to 4 years, 5 to 10 years

Phenylketonuria (PKU) screening for newborns

Sexually transmitted infection (STI) prevention counseling and screening for adolescents at higher risk

Tuberculin testing for children at higher risk of tuberculosis ages: 0 to 11 months, 1 to 4 years, 5 to 10 years, 11 to 14 years, 15 to 17 years

Vision screening for all children

USELESS TESTS

Scientific and professional organizations have determined the following tests to have no benefit or to be outright harmful.[1,2]

Cancer Screenings
Cancer screening for patients with chronic kidney disease (CKD) receiving dialysis

Cervical cancer screening for women over age 65

Colorectal cancer screening for adults over age 85

Prostate-specific antigen (PSA) testing for men over age 75

Diagnostic and Preventive Testing
Bone mineral density testing at frequent intervals for patients with osteoporosis

Homocysteine testing for cardiovascular disease

Hypercoagulability testing for patients

with deep vein thrombosis

Parathyroid hormone (PTH) measurement for patients with stage 1–3 CKD

Preoperative Testing

Preoperative chest radiography

Preoperative echocardiography

Preoperative pulmonary function testing (PFT)

Preoperative stress testing

Imaging

Computed tomography (CT) of the sinuses for uncomplicated acute rhinosinusitis for patients with sinusitis diagnosis

Head imaging in the evaluation of syncope

Head imaging for uncomplicated headache

Electroencephalogram (EEG) for headaches

Back imaging for patients with nonspecific low back pain

Screening for carotid artery disease in asymptomatic adults

Screening for carotid artery disease for syncope

Cardiovascular Testing and Procedures

Carotid endarterectomy in asymptomatic patients

Inferior vena cava filters for the prevention of pulmonary embolism

Percutaneous coronary intervention with balloon angioplasty or stent placement for stable coronary disease for patients with ischemic heart disease (IHD)

Renal artery angioplasty or stenting for patients with hypertension

Stress testing for stable coronary disease for patients with IHD

Other Surgery

Vertebroplasty or kyphoplasty for osteoporotic vertebral fractures in patients with osteoporosis

Arthroscopic surgery for knee osteoarthritis for patients with arthritis

MEDICATIONS GIVEN BEFORE, DURING, AND AFTER PROCEDURES

Before Procedures

Large-spectrum antibiotic — for example, Ancef or cefazolin

During Procedures

Barbiturates and/or benzodiazepines: Medication used to relax a patient just prior to surgery commencing — for example, Valium or Versed

Local anesthesia: Medication injected into the skin to numb or block pain in a specific site

Regional anesthesia: Medication injected into a cluster of nerves to numb the part of the body that is undergoing the procedure — for example, an epidural during labor and delivery

General anesthesia: Medication given via IV to put the patient to sleep and suppress pain throughout the entire body — for example, Propofol; sometimes a temporary paralytic, such as Succinylcholine

After Procedures
Pain management:

Opioids: Examples: Duramorph (morphine), Dilaudid (hydromorphone) — typically given in tab form as Lorotab or Percocet upon discharge to manage pain (see page 264 for a discussion of opioids)

Analgesic pain management: Examples: Tylenol (acetaminophen), ibuprofen

Anticoagulants: Used to prevent clotting, a major risk of surgery as the body responds to injury by making platelets to reduce bleeding — for example, Coumadin (warfarin), Heparin, Lovenox (enoxaparin)

Additional
Stool softener: To counteract opioid-induced constipation and sluggish GI system after surgery — for example, Colace (docusate sodium) or Senokot

Acid reducer: Famotidine

Anti-nausea medications: Zofran, Phenergan

OPIOID TYPES
AND SIDE EFFECTS

Types of Opioids
Codeine (only available in generic form)
Fentanyl (Abstral, Actiq, Duragesic, Fentora, Onsolis)
Hydrocodone (Hysingla ER, Zohydro ER)
Hydrocodone and acetaminophen (Lorcet, Lortab, Norco, Vicodin)
Hydromorphone (Dilaudid, Exalgo)
Meperidine (Demerol)
Methadone (Dolophine, Methadose)
Morphine (Kadian, MS Contin, Morpha-Bond ER)
Oxycodone (Oxaydo, OxyContin)
Oxycodone and acetaminophen (Percocet, Roxicet)
Oxycodone and naloxone

Side Effects
Constipation (most common)
Dizziness
Nausea (highly common)

Sedation
Respiratory depression (most dangerous)

NOTES

Preface

1. Philip F. Stahel, Todd F. VanderHeiden, and Fernando J. Kim, "Why Do Surgeons Continue to Perform Unnecessary Surgery?," *Patient Safety in Surgery* 11, no. 1 (January 2017), http://www.ncbi.nlm.nih. gov/pmc/articles/PMC5234149.

Chapter 2: Unlearn What You Know About Being a Patient

1. David K. C. Cooper and Denton A. Cooley, "Christiaan Neethling Barnard, 1922–2001," *Journal of the American Heart Association* 104 (2001): 2756–57, https:// www.ahajournals.org/doi/pdf/10.1161/ hc4801.100999.
2. *Healthy People 2010* (Washington, DC: US Department of Health and Human Services, Office of Disease Prevention and

Health Promotion, 2000) and S. C. Ratzan, R. M. Parker, introduction to *National Library of Medicine Current Bibliographies in Medicine: Health Literacy,* eds. C. R. Selden, M. Zorn, S. C. Ratzan, R. M. Parker (Bethesda, MD: National Institutes of Health, U.S. Department of Health and Human Services, 2000).

Chapter 3: Appoint a Team

1. The research in this area is relatively new and is limited to physicians, so I'll be talking about doctors specifically in this section, not nurse practitioners or physician assistants.
2. N. Lurie et al., "Preventive Care for Women. Does the Sex of the Physician Matter?," *New England Journal of Medicine* 329, no. 7 (August 1993): 478–82.
3. E. Frank and L. K. Harvey, "Prevention Advice Rates of Women and Men Physicians," *Archives of Family Medicine* 5, no. 4 (April 1996): 215–19.
4. N. Lurie et al., "Preventive Care for Women."
5. Franca Pizzini, "Communication Hierarchies in Humour: Gender Differences in the Obstetrical/Gynaecological Setting,"

Discourse & Society 2, no. 4 (1991): 477–88.

6. R. Borgès Da Silva, V. Martel, and R. Blais, "Qualité et Productivité dans les Groupes de Médecine de Famille: Qui Sont les Meilleurs? Les Hommes ou les Femmes?," *Revue d'Épidémiologie et de Santé Publique* 61, supplement 4 (October 2013): S210–S211.

7. Christopher J. D. Wallis et al., "Comparison of Postoperative Outcomes among Patients Treated by Male and Female Surgeons: A Population Based Matched Cohort Study," *BMJ* 359 (2017), http://www.doi.org/10.1136/bmj.j4366.

8. Philip M. Eskew and Kathleen Klink, "Direct Primary Care: Practice Distribution and Cost Across the Nation," *Journal of the American Board of Family Medicine* 28, no. 6 (2015): 793–801.

9. Tami L. Mark, Katharine R. Levit, and Jeffrey A. Buck, "Datapoints: Psychotropic Drug Prescriptions by Medical Specialty," *Psychiatric Services* 60, no. 9 (September 2009): 1167.

10. Reza Nemati et al., "Deposition and Hydrolysis of Serine Dipeptide Lipids of Bacteroidetes Bacteria in Human Arteries: Relationship to Atherosclerosis," *Journal of Lipid Research* 58, no. 10 (October

11. A. Haerian-Ardakani et al., "Relationship between Maternal Periodontal Disease and Low Birth Weight Babies," *Iranian Journal of Reproductive Medicine* 11, no. 8 (2013): 625–30.

Chapter 8: When Something Is Wrong

1. Lenny Bernstein, "20 Percent of Patients with Serious Conditions Are First Misdiagnosed, Study Says," *Washington Post,* April 4, 2017, https://www.washingtonpost .com/national/health-science/20-percent -of-patients-with-serious-conditions-are -first-misdiagnosed-study-says/2017/04/ 03/e386982a-189f-11e7-9887-1a5314b56 a08_story.html?utm_term=.878627c6 c92c.

Chapter 9: Navigating Touchy Territory

1. "Is It Time to Drop the 'Complete the Course' Message for Antibiotics?," University of Oxford, July 27, 2017, http://www .ox.ac.uk/news/2017-07-27-it-time-drop -'complete-course'-message-antibiotics.
2. L. E. Markowitz et al., "Reduction in Human Papillomavirus (HPV) Prevalence among Young Women Following HPV Vac-

cine Introduction in the United States, National Health and Nutrition Examination Surveys, 2003–2010," *Journal of Infectious Diseases* 208, no. 3 (2013): 385–93.

3. S. Reagan-Steiner et al., "National, Regional, State, and Selected Local Area Vaccination Coverage among Adolescents Aged 13–17 years — United States, 2015," *Morbidity and Mortality Weekly Report* 65 (2016): 850–58, http://dx.doi.org/10.15585/mmwr.mm6533a4; Markowitz, "Reduction in Human Papillomavirus."

4. R. P. Wildman, P. Muntner, and K. Reynolds, "The Obese without Cardiometabolic Risk Factor Clustering and the Normal Weight with Cardiometabolic Risk Factor Clustering," *Archives of Internal Medicine* 168, no. 15 (2008): 1617–24, http://www.jamanetwork.com/journals/jamainternalmedicine/fullarticle/770362.

Chapter 14: ER vs. Urgent Care vs. Wait Until Monday

1. Maggie Fox, "Major Insurance Company's Payment Decision Angers ER Doctors," NBC News, June 3, 2017, https://www.nbcnews.com/health/health-news/major-insurance-company-s-payment-decision-angers-er-doctors-n767766.

Chapter 17: Choosing If, Where, and Who

1. Philip F. Stahel, Todd F. VanderHeiden, and Fernando J. Kim, "Why Do Surgeons Continue to Perform Unnecessary Surgery?," *Patient Safety in Surgery* 11 (2017): 1. *BMC.* Web. October 15, 2018.
2. Velma L. Payne et al., "Patient-Initiated Second Opinions: Systematic Review of Characteristics and Impact on Diagnosis, Treatment, and Satisfaction," *Mayo Clinic Proceedings* 89, no. 5 (2014): 687–96, http://www.mayoclinicproceedings.org/article/S0025-6196%2814%2900245-6/fulltext.

Chapter 20: How to Be Vigilant

1. Amanda Gardner, "Surgery Mix-Ups Surprisingly Common," Health.com, October 18, 2010, http://www.cnn.com/2010/HEALTH/10/18/health.surgery.mixups.common.

Chapter 22: When It's Your Kid

1. Vaccine Education Center at the Children's Hospital of Philadelphia, "Aluminum in Vaccines: What You Should Know," *Q&A* 5 (2014), https://media.chop.edu/

data/files/pdfs/vaccine-education-center
-aluminum.pdf.

Part IX: When You're Not a Straight White Male

1. Lu Chen and Christopher I. Li, "Racial Disparities in Breast Cancer Diagnosis and Treatment by Hormone Receptor and HER2 Status," *Cancer Epidemiology, Biomarkers & Prevention* 11 (October 2015): DOI: 10.1158/1055-9965.EPI-15-0293.
2. Maya Dusenbery, *Doing Harm: The Truth About How Bad Medicine and Lazy Science Leave Women Dismissed, Misdiagnosed, and Sick* (New York: HarperOne, 2018), pages throughout.

Chapter 24: The Female Patient

1. A. Parekh et al., "Adverse Effects in Women: Implications for Drug Development and Regulatory Policies," *Expert Review of Clinical Pharmacology* 4, no. 4 (July 2011): 453–466, DOI: 10.1586/ecp.11.29.
2. K. L. Calderone, "The Influence of Gender on the Frequency of Pain and Sedative Medication Administered to Postoperative Patients," *Sex Roles* 23, no.

11–12 (December 1990): 713, https://doi
.org/10.1007/BF00289259.
3. J. L. Clarke et al., "The Diagnosis of
CAD in Women: Addressing the Unmet
Need — A Report from the National
Expert Roundtable Meeting," *Population
Health Management* 18, no. 2 (April 2015):
86–92.

Chapter 25: When You're Having a Baby

1. M. F. MacDorman et al., "Recent In-
creases in the U.S. Maternal Mortality
Rate: Disentangling Trends from Measure-
ment Issue," *Obstetrics and Gynecology*
128, no. 3 (September 2016): 447–55.
2. S. Reagan-Steiner et al., "National,
Regional, State, and Selected Local Area
Vaccination Coverage among Adolescents
Aged 13–17 Years." Markowitz, "Reduc-
tion in Human Papillomavirus."
3. M. Johantgen et al., "Comparison of
Labor and Delivery Care Provided by
Certified Nurse-Midwives and Physicians:
A Systematic Review, 1990 to 2008,"
Women's Health Issues 22 (2012): e73–
81; J. Sandall et al., "Midwife-Led Conti-
nuity Models Versus Other Models of
Care for Childbearing Women," *Cochrane
Database of Systematic Reviews,*

CD004667 (2016); K. Sutcliffe et al., "Comparing Midwife-Led and Doctor-Led Maternity Care: A Systematic Review of Reviews," *Journal of Advanced Nursing* 68, no. 11 (2012): 2376–86.

4. J. Sandall et al., "Midwife-Led Continuity Models"; K. Sutcliffe et al., "Comparing Midwife-Led and Doctor-Led Maternity Care."

5. M. Johantgen et al., "Comparison of Labor and Delivery Care."

Chapter 27: Implicit Bias and Systemic Oppression

1. "Fact Sheets: Disparities," Indian Health Service, accessed January 17, 2019, https://www.ihs.gov/newsroom/factsheets/disparities/.

2. E. K. Spanakis and S. H. Golden, "Race/Ethnic Difference in Diabetes and Diabetic Complications." *Current Diabetes Reports* 13, no. 6 (December 2013): 814–23.

3. Eileen Patten, "Racial, Gender Wage Gaps Persist in U.S. Despite Some Progress," Pew Research Center, July 1, 2016, http://www.pewresearch.org/fact-tank/2016/07/01/racial-gender-wage-gaps-persist-in-u-s-despite-some-progress/.

4. K. M. Hoffman et al., "Racial Bias in

Pain Assessment and Treatment Recommendations, and False Beliefs About Biological Differences Between Blacks and Whites," *Proceedings of the National Academy of Sciences of the United States of America* 113, no. 16 (April 2016): 4296–4301.

5. M. K. Goyal et al., "Racial Disparities in Pain Management of Children with Appendicitis in Emergency Departments," *JAMA Pediatrics* 169, no. 11 (November 2015): 996–1002.
6. K. M. Hoffman et al., "Racial Bias in Pain Assessment and Treatment Recommendations," 4296–4301.
7. American Medical Association Principles of Medical Ethics: I, IV, V, VIII, IX.

Chapter 28: How to Deal with Insurance

1. Nick Tate, "4 in 5 Medical Bills Contain Errors: Here's What You Can Do," NewsMax Health, August 7, 2017, https://www.newsmax.com/health/health-news/medical-bill-error-mistake/2017/08/04/id/805882/.

Chapter 29: Big Pharma and the FDA

1. C. DeJong et al., "Pharmaceutical Industry–Sponsored Meals and Physician Prescribing Patterns for Medicare Beneficiaries," *JAMA Internal Medicine* 176, no. 8 (2016): 1114–22, doi:10.1001/jamaint -ernmed.2016.2765.
2. Aaron E. Carroll, "Heart Stents Are Useless for Most Stable Patients. They're Still Widely Used," Upshot (blog), *New York Times,* February 12, 2018, http://www .nytimes.com/2018/02/12/upshot/heart -stents-are-useless-for-most-stable -patients-theyre-still-widely-used.html; Kathleen Stergiopoulos and David L. Brown, "Initial Coronary Stent Implantation with Medical Therapy vs. Medical Therapy Alone for Stable Coronary Artery Disease: Meta-Analysis of Randomized Controlled Trials," *Archives of Internal Medicine* 172, no. 4 (2012): 312–19, http://www.jamanetwork.com/journals/ jamainternalmedicine/fullarticle/1108733.
3. J. J. Darrow, "Explaining the Absence of Surgical Procedure Regulation," *Cornell Journal of Law and Public Policy* 27, no. 1 (2017): 189–206; Stahel, VanderHeiden, and Kim, "Why Do Surgeons Continue to Perform Unnecessary Surgery?"; Freder-

ick A. Masoudi et al., "Trends in U.S. Cardiovascular Care: 2016 Report from 4 ACC National Cardiovascular Data Registries," *Journal of the American College of Cardiology* (2016), http://www.onlinejacc .org/content/early/2016/12/20/j.jacc.2016 .12.005.

Appendix: Medical Jargon

1. William C. Shiel Jr., "Common Medical Abbreviations and Acronyms List," MedicineNet, ed. Melissa Conrad Stöppler, https://www.medicinenet.com/common _medical_abbreviations_and_terms/article .htm#medical_abbreviations_what_do _they_mean.

Appendix: Useless Tests

1. Atul Gawande, "Overkill," *The New Yorker,* May 11, 2015, https://www .newyorker.com/magazine/2015/05/11/ overkill-atul-gawande.
2. Aaron L. Schwartz et al., "Measuring Low-Value Care in Medicare," *JAMA Internal Medicine* 174, no. 7 (2014): 1067–76, http://www.jamanetwork.com/journals/ jamainternalmedicine/fullarticle/1868536.

ABOUT THE AUTHOR

Sana Goldberg liaises between academia and clinical practice. She has worked with a diversity of patients across settings from the perspective of researcher, social worker, nurse, and provider. A public health advocate, she's presented at World Congress, TEDx Harvard, the Society for Neuroscience, and OPHA, with work published in *Neuropharmacology,* the *European Journal of Neuroscience,* and forthcoming in *The Atlantic.* She is a member of the International Honor Society of Nursing and the founder of Nightingale, a movement of story, art, and activism for health equity. She practices in New Haven, Connecticut, while pursuing graduate studies at Yale.

The employees of Thorndike Press hope you have enjoyed this Large Print book. All our Thorndike, Wheeler, and Kennebec Large Print titles are designed for easy reading, and all our books are made to last. Other Thorndike Press Large Print books are available at your library, through selected bookstores, or directly from us.

For information about titles, please call:
  (800) 223-1244

or visit our website at:
  gale.com/thorndike

To share your comments, please write:
  Publisher
  Thorndike Press
  10 Water St., Suite 310
  Waterville, ME 04901